Geriatric Nutrition & Diet Therapy

3rd Edition

Marie Jaffe, R.N., M.S. (deceased)
Revision Author: Beth Holthausen, M.S., R.D.

Contributor:
James Hobbs, R.Ph.

A SKIDMORE-ROTH PUBLICATION

SR
PUBLISHING

Publisher: Linda Skidmore-Roth
Developmental Editor: Molly Sullivan, B.A.
Copy Editor: Kathryn Head, B.A.
Cover Design: Barbara Barr, Visual Impact
Typesetting: Gary Grudowski
Printing: Gilliland Printing

Notice: The author and publisher of this volume have taken care to make certain that all information is correct and compatible with standards generally accepted at the time of publication. Because the science of nursing is constantly changing and expanding, new techniques and concepts are continually implemented. Therefore, the reader is encouraged to stay abreast of new developments in the nursing field and to be aware that policies vary according to the guidelines of each school or institution.

Jaffe, Marie (Deceased)
Geriatric Nutrition and Diet Therapy

ISBN 1-56930-096-8
1. Nursing Handbooks, Manuals
2. Medical Handbooks, Manuals

Skidmore-Roth Publishing, Inc.
400 Inverness Dr. South
Suite 260
Englewood, CO 80112
1 (800) 825-3150
www.skidmore-roth.com

INTRODUCTION

The older adult has special nutritional needs and requirements that differ from those during other stages of life. Although no specific requirements are determined for the above 50 age group, many factors influence the nutritional status and dictate the food and fluid intake needs of these individuals. Some of these factors include: physiologic changes, physical handicaps, multiple medications, chronic illness, life-long dietary habits, economics, and psychological problems. The nutritional status of older adults can be affected by one or more of the above determinants with the only commonality among the group being chronological age.

Physiologic aging changes associated with nutritional problems of the older adult include reduced circulatory and respiratory function (movement of nutrients and oxygen to all body tissues), decreased ingestion (chewing, swallowing, gustatory and olfactory perceptions, inability to feed self), decreased digestion (chewing, enzyme/other secretions and gastrointestinal motility reduction), decreased metabolic rate and excretion (constipation or diarrhea, fluid and electrolyte imbalance). Physical handicaps that influence nutrition include decreased visual acuity (cataracts), weakness, and inability to manipulate eating utensils (poor coordination, muscle atrophy, muscle rigidity, joint pain). Medications include those that impair the level of consciousness, increase or decrease appetite, or interact with nutrients. Chronic illnesses common to the older adult that affect nutrition include diabetes mellitus, arthritis, heart disease, hypertension, dementia, anemia, chronic renal failure, chronic obstructive pulmonary disease, and malignant tumor. Life-long dietary habits developed over many years determine food preferences and can place an older adult in a state of deficiency for one or more nutrients. This can also result in noncompliant behavior, lack of acceptance of dietary inclusions, or restrictions related to a chronic illness. Economic factors include the inability to purchase necessary nutritional foods. Many older adults have fixed low incomes, some below the poverty line, that can severely restrict the type of foods selected. Psychologic problems that most affect nutritional status are the loss of persons or objects, loneliness and isolation, refusal to eat, fear for personal safety, confusion, apathy, depression, and suicidal tendency.

To assist in the improvement of nutrition, the government grants money to each state to finance low cost nutritional programs for individuals over 60 years of age. Some examples are community programs such as Meals-on-Wheels (a home delivered program for the homebound) and Congregrate Meals Program (central kitchen providing a daily hot meal and socialization). The Food Stamp Program offers stamps that are redeemed for food to those with low incomes.

This book is dedicated to the ever-increasing older adult population who consider eating a pleasure as well as a necessity for a healthy existence. It has been conceived and developed to acquaint nurses with changes in the aging process affecting nutritional and fluid needs. It can be used by the independent older adult, or health professionals and adjunct staff responsible for the nutritional needs of the partially or totally dependent individual. Because of its nursing perspective, it can be incorporated into home care plans, although its approach reflects the nutritional guidance and integration needed for the care of the older adult in long-term or alternative care facilities. It is limited to a handbook style and format to be used as an adjunct to more in-depth, comprehensive nutritional resources for information, if needed, for dietary changes or maintenance.

My thanks to Linda Skidmore-Roth for the opportunity to revise this book and the staff of Skidmore-Roth Publishing Co. for their willing and cordial assistance in its development and completion.

Marie S. Jaffe (Deceased)

TABLE OF CONTENTS

CHAPTER I
GASTROINTESTINAL SYSTEM

A.   Anatomy and Physiology
B.   Changes Related to Aging Process
C.   Flow Sheets: Ingestion, Digestion,
      Absorption, Elimination

ANATOMY AND PHYSIOLOGY

The gastrointestinal (GI) system, also known as the alimentary tract, consists of a hollow tubular structure that begins with the oral cavity and ends with the anus, plus the associated organs that provide the body with the necessary nutrients and substances for life. Nutrients, waste, vitamins, minerals, and electrolytes are received by the tract and are moved through it at a rate regulated by motility, secretions, and absorption. (See Fig. 1.1.) Innervation of the system is accomplished by the autonomic nervous system; the parasympathetic branch is excitatory and increases peristalsis, and the sympathetic branch is inhibitory and decreases peristalsis. The primary function of the system is to supply nutrients to cells, tissues, and organs by ingestion (eating food and drinking fluids), movement of foods and fluid through the tract (peristalsis), digestion (breaking down of food by its secretions), absorption (transfer of nutrients into the circulation), and elimination (excretion of solid waste). The system includes the mouth, teeth, tongue, salivary glands (parotid, submaxillary, sublingual), pharynx, esophagus, stomach, small intestine (duodenum, jejunum, ileum), pancreas, liver, gallbladder, and large intestine (ascending, transverse, descending colon, rectum, anus).

The components of the system and their functions are as follows:

1. **Oral cavity:** Receives food (bolus) and begins preparation for absorption. The oral cavity contains: teeth to masticate the food to sizes appropriate for swallowing (deglutition); the tongue which contains taste buds (gustatory perception) and positions food for swallowing; muscles for chewing and moving food; a large surface area on which enzymes can act; salivary glands that secrete 1,000-1,500 mL/day of saliva, including salivary amylase (ptyalin) to moisten the food and begin the digestion of starches by converting them to maltose.

2. **Pharynx:** Closes the trachea as it moves food into the esophagus.

3. **Esophagus:** A 10 inch tube that connects the pharynx with the stomach and provides a passageway for the food. Contains mucus secreting glands that lubricate the bolus as it passes through the tube by peristaltic waves. It is positioned behind the trachea and contains a sphincter (pressure zone) at its distal end about 2 inches above the entry into the stomach (cardiac sphincter). This entry remains closed unless decreased pressure relaxes the sphincter, allowing the passage of food into the stomach. This area provides a barrier to protect the esophageal mucosa from the backflow of gastric secretions (gastric reflux) as pressure is increased.

4. **Stomach:** A hollow, pouch-like organ that stores the food early in the digestive process. It has the capacity of 1,500 mL and, in addition to storage, mixes and liquifies the food and controls passage of the food into the duodenum by the pyloric sphincter at the stomach's distal end. Glands in the stomach secrete pepsinogen (chief cells that digest protein), hydrochloric acid, the intrinsic factor glycoprotein (parietal cells), and mucus (mucous neck cells). About 2,000 mL/day of gastric juices are secreted to mix with food to form chyme, which is propelled into the duodenum through the pyloric sphincter in small amounts by peristalsis (every 15-25 seconds). The source of the blood supply to the stomach is the celiac artery. Gastric veins that connect and terminate in the portal vein drain the venous blood. Gastrin is the hormone secreted by the antrum of the stomach and duodenum that stimulates the secretion of pepsin, hydrochloric acid, and pancreatic enzymes, and increases the flow of bile and smooth muscle contractions. Enzymes in gastric juices include gastric lipase, and pepsin I, II, III. The digestion of carbohydrates begun in the oral cavity continues in the stomach and protein digestion begins. There is no significant fat digestion in the stomach.

5. **Small intestine:** This portion of the tract is about 22 feet long and consists of the duodenum (<1 foot), jejunum (8 feet), and ileum (12 feet). It receives the chyme and

further mixes and breaks it down as it is propelled toward the large intestine. The chyme remains in the small intestine for up to 10 hours. About 3,000 mL/day of digestive enzymes (maltase, lactase, dextrinase, sucrase, intestinal lipase, and the peptidases) are secreted, as well as hormones which control the secretions and motility (gastrin, secretin, cholecystokinin, gastric inhibitory peptide, motilin, and somatostatin). These assist with the digestion and absorption of proteins, carbohydrates, and fats that are taking place in this part of the tract. The peristaltic activity produces from 9-12 movements/minute and serves to mix the chyme with the enzymes and bile responsible for the breakdown of the substances to simpler forms. Absorption then takes place by diffusion through the wall to the capillary beds. The sources of the blood supply to the small intestine are the superior mesenteric and hepatic arteries. The superior mesenteric vein that connects with the inferior mesenteric vein and empties into the portal vein and liver drains the venous blood. The circulatory system transports the diffused nutrients to the body cells.

6. **Liver/Gallbladder:** The liver is the largest gland in the body, weighing about 3 pounds and secreting about 1,000 mL bile/day. Its metabolic functions include the production and secretion of bile; the metabolism of protein, carbohydrates, and fats; the detoxification of drugs; steroid metabolism; and the storage of glucose, vitamins, fatty acids, amino acids, and minerals. Important components of bile are bile salts that assist in the breakdown of fat globules and the absorption of fatty acids, monoglycerides, cholesterol, and lipids in the intestine. The gallbladder is a pear-shaped organ that concentrates and stores bile. It has a capacity of 100-150 mL and receives the bile from the liver via the hepatic ducts. Bile is necessary for fat digestion. When fatty foods enter the small intestine, cholecystokinin is released and the gallbladder contracts. This allows the bile to move through the cystic duct into the duodenum via its connection to the common bile duct. At the same

time, a valve at the end of the common bile duct (sphincter of Oddi) opens in the presence of fat in the intestine, allowing the bile to flow into the duodenum. Bile is eventually reduced to urobilinogen by bacterial action, and eliminated in the feces.

7. **Pancreas:** This gland has the capacity to produce 1,500-3,000 mL of digestive juices per day. It contains exocrine acini cells which secrete the digestive juices, pancreatic amylase for carbohydrate metabolism; lipase for fat metabolism, and trypsin for protein metabolism. They empty into the duodenum via the common bile duct. The site where a duct from the pancreas connects with the common bile duct is called the ampulla of Vater. The pancreas also contains endocrine islet beta cells which secrete insulin, and alpha cells that secrete glucagon. These substances are involved in glucose metabolism. Diabetes mellitus occurs when there is an imbalance between insulin availability and insulin need and alters carbohydrate, protein and fat metabolism.

8. **Large intestine:** Also known as the colon, this portion of the tract is 5 feet long and consists of the cecum, ascending colon, transverse colon, descending colon, sigmoid colon, rectum, and anus. Its major functions are the absorption of water and electrolytes (sodium and chloride), allowing the formation of feces, and the elimination of feces from the body. It secretes mucus to lubricate and promote movement of the feces through the bowel and protects the mucosa from irritation or injury. Bicarbonate is secreted to assist in neutralizing the acidic end-products of bacterial action. The source of the blood supply are the superior and inferior mesen-teric, and rectal arteries. The blood is drained by the superior and inferior mesenteric veins to the portal vein and liver. As the chyme passes through the ileocecal valve to the cecum and distends the bowel, the walls contract and peristaltic waves move the mass through the bowel. Feces consists of water and solids containing food by-products, enzymes, bile pigments, mucus, and salts. Defecation occurs as the rectum becomes

distended and increases the pressure that, in turn, relaxes the internal and external sphincter muscles.

The Gastrointestinal System (Fig. 1.1)

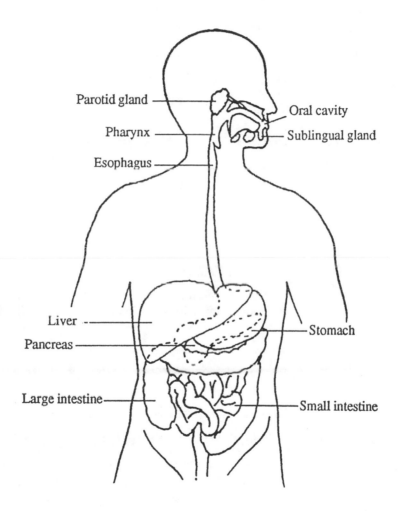

Location of Gastrointestinal Organs

Right Upper Quadrant
Gallbladder
Duodenum
Head of pancreas
Lobe of liver
Upper part of kidney
Pylorus of stomach

Left Upper Quadrant
Lobe of liver
Spleen
Kidney
Stomach
Body of pancreas
Left transverse colon

Right Lower Quadrant
Lower part of kidney
Cecum
Ascending colon
Appendix

Left Lower Quadrant
Sigmoid colon
Descending colon

CENTRAL ABDOMEN
Small intestine
(Duodenum, Jejunum, Ileum)

Gastrointestinal Hormones

Hormone	Site	Stimulus	Action
Gastrin	Antial mucosa of stomach	Antial distention; vagal stimulus; partially digested proteins in the antrum	Stimulates gastric secretion and mobility

Gastrointestinal Digestive Substances*—

Hormones

Hormone	Site	Stimulus	Action
Cholecystokinin (CCK)	Duodenum, Jejunum	Fats in duodenum	Stimulates gallbladder contraction to release bile, small bowel motility, secretions of pepsin, pancreatic juice and digestive enzymes
Secretin	Duodenal mucosa	Fats and sugars in duodenum gut acidity	Inhibits gastric motility and gastric acid secretion, relaxes sphincter of Oddi
Gastric inhibitory peptide (GIP)	Duodenum, Jejunum	Glucose, fat and amino acid in duodenum	Inhibits gastric acid and pepsin secretions, stimulates intestinal juice and insulin secretions
Motilin	Upper small intestine	Duodenal alkalinity	Decreases gastric emptying and stimulates gut mobility

Gastrointestinal Digestive Substances*—

Hormones

Hormone	Site	Stimulus	Action
Somatostatin	Stomach, Duodenum, Pancreas	Secretin, glucagon, acid in duodenum	Inhibits gastrin, motilin, gastric acid, pancreatic enzyme, bicarbonate secretions, gallbladder, stomach, and intestinal motility

Enzymes

Enzyme	Site	Action	End-Product
Pytalin (salivary amylase)	Submaxillary, Parotid glands	Starch	Polysaccharides into disaccharides
Pepsins (I, II, III)	Stomach chief cells	Proteins	Polypeptides
Gastric lipase	Stomach	Triglycerides	Glycerides
Pancreatic amylase	Pancreas	Starch	Polysaccharides into disaccharides
Pancreatic lipase	Pancreas	Triglycerides	Monoglycerides
Trypsin	Pancreas	Polypeptides	Split chains
Enterokinase	Duodenum	Trypsinogen	Trypsin
Intestinal lipase	Intestines	Splits fats	Glycerol, fatty acids
Maltase	Intestines	Maltose	Glucose
Lactase	Intestines	Lactose	Glucose and galactose

Enzymes

Enzyme	Site	Action	End-Product
Sucrase	Intestines	Sucrose	Glucose and fructose
Aminopeptidase	Intestines	Polypeptides	Peptides
Dipeptidase	Intestines	Dipeptides	Amino acids

Absorption Sites

Intake	Site
Protein	Jejunum
Carbohydrate	Jejunum
Fat	Jejunum
Vitamins	Duodenum (B_{12} in ileum)
Minerals	Small intestine
Water	Small and large intestine

Adapted with permission from Black, JM and Matassarin-Jacobs, E. Luckhamm and Sorenson's Medical-Surgical Nursing (4th ed.). WB Saunders, Philadelphia, 1993, pp. 1550-1551.

Gastrointestinal Changes Related to the Aging Process

Alterations in the digestive process resulting from the aging process include physiologic changes involving secretion, reduction of nutrients, absorption, motility, and transport. Digestive disorders and eating problems tend to be more prevalent in the older adult, at times because of chronic disease rather than changes associated with the aging process. Nervous system changes may include sensory and motor losses affecting peripheral nerve conduction; parasympathetic and sympathic functions affecting intestinal motility and enzymatic release; and decreased vasomotor reponse affecting ingestion. The most common complaints of the older adult involve the gastrointestinal system, beginning with the mouth (teeth, chewing, swallowing) and ending with the process of elimination (constipation). The disorders most commonly associated with the aging population affecting this system are obstructive processes, absorption problems, vascular abnormalities, and neurologic changes.

Organ Structure/Anatomy

1. Thinning of tooth enamel causing teeth to become brittle.

2. Wearing down and loss of teeth causing chewing impairment.

3. Bone loss in oral structures causing difficulty in fitting dentures and decreased tooth support.

4. Thinning and drying of oral epithelium allowing for irritation and damage to the mucous membrane.

5. Increasing body fat and decreasing lean body mass; changes in fat distribution with decreases in extremities and increases in abdomen and hips.

6. Gradually decreasing weight with decreases in women occurring more slowly than in men.

7. Decreasing subcutaneous tissue causing difficulty in environmental temperature adjustments.

8. Decreasing number and size of liver cells causing a reduction in weight and mass of liver; pancreatic atrophy causing a decrease in exocrine cells for enzyme production.

9. Alveolar degeneration and obstruction of ducts of the pancreas causing the blocking of secretions.

10. Decreasing mucosal surface area of small intestine causing altered absorption of nutrients.

11. Atrophy of mucosa, muscle layers, arteriolar sclerosis, delay in peripheral nerve transmission of the colon causing constipation or fecal incontinence.

12. Weakening of abdominal and pelvic muscles causing difficulty in defecation.

Physiologic Function

1. Reduction in saliva production causing dry mouth and risk for breakdown of oral mucosa.

2. Taste and smell dysfunction causing altered taste perception and a reduced food intake.

3. Changing pH of saliva from acid to alkaline causing increasing tendency for tooth decay.

4. Decreasing gag reflex causing swallowing difficulty.

5. Decreasing peristaltic activity of the esophagus and relaxation of the smooth muscle of lower esophagus causing delayed emptying, dilitation, and reflux.

6. Decreasing pepsin, hydrochloric acid secretions, and intrinsic factor by stomach; a thinning mucosa, atrophic changes in the mucosa, and increased rate of cell loss causing reduced absorption of vitamin B_1, B_2, B_{12}.

7. Decreasing gastric motility causing delayed gastric emptying and possibly delayed absorption of medications.

8. Reduction in ptyalin with reduced saliva, and reduction in lipase and mucin secretions by stomach causing delay in digestive processes.

9. Decreasing metabolic rate causing weight gain.

10. Decreasing hepatic enzyme concentration causing a reduced enzyme response to drug detoxification and metabolism.

11. Thicker bile, containing higher cholesterol concentrations and reduced volume with more difficult emptying causing biliary tract disease (cholelithiasis) and obstruction; decreasing fat soluble vitamin absorption by bile.

12. Decreasing secretion of amylase, lipase, and trypsin by the pancreas causing impaired digestion of lipids and splitting of large polypeptides into peptides that are acted upon in a singular fashion by the small intestine.

13. Decreasing absorption of nutrients by the small intestine and reduction in the efficiency of the transport mechanism.

14. Decreasing enzyme secretion causing an increase in time required for digestion and reduction in bacterial flora in the large intestine.

15. Decreasing bowel motility, gastrocolic reflex, voluntary contraction of the external sphincter and amount of feces, contributing to constipation or fecal incontinence.

16. Vasculature of digestive tract (atherosclerosis) causing decreasing blood supply of nutrients to bowel and possible tissue injury.

17. Decreasing hunger contractions causing delayed gastric emptying.

18. Decreasing muscle tone and peristalsis of the bowel causing constipation and risk for obstruction.

19. Increasing swallowing of air when eating causing distention and eructation.

Physiology Flow Sheet (Figure 1.2)

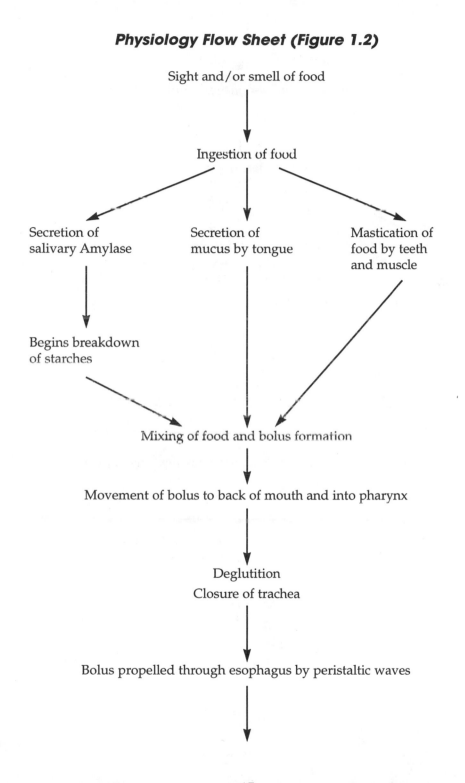

Sight and/or smell of food

Ingestion of food

Secretion of salivary Amylase

Secretion of mucus by tongue

Mastication of food by teeth and muscle

Begins breakdown of starches

Mixing of food and bolus formation

Movement of bolus to back of mouth and into pharynx

Deglutition
Closure of trachea

Bolus propelled through esophagus by peristaltic waves

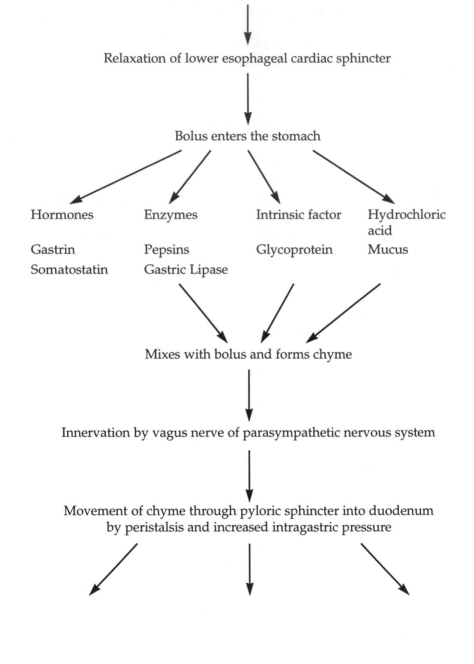

Relaxation of lower esophageal cardiac sphincter

Bolus enters the stomach

Hormones   Enzymes   Intrinsic factor   Hydrochloric acid

Gastrin   Pepsins   Glycoprotein   Mucus
Somatostatin   Gastric Lipase

Mixes with bolus and forms chyme

Innervation by vagus nerve of parasympathetic nervous system

Movement of chyme through pyloric sphincter into duodenum
by peristalsis and increased intragastric pressure

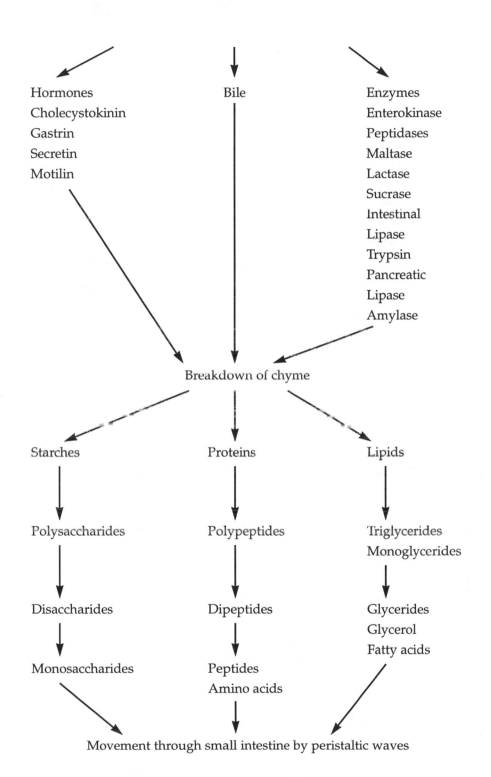

Hormones
Cholecystokinin
Gastrin
Secretin
Motilin

Bile

Enzymes
Enterokinase
Peptidases
Maltase
Lactase
Sucrase
Intestinal
Lipase
Trypsin
Pancreatic
Lipase
Amylase

Breakdown of chyme

Starches

Polysaccharides

Disaccharides

Monosaccharides

Proteins

Polypeptides

Dipeptides

Peptides
Amino acids

Lipids

Triglycerides
Monoglycerides

Glycerides
Glycerol
Fatty acids

Movement through small intestine by peristaltic waves

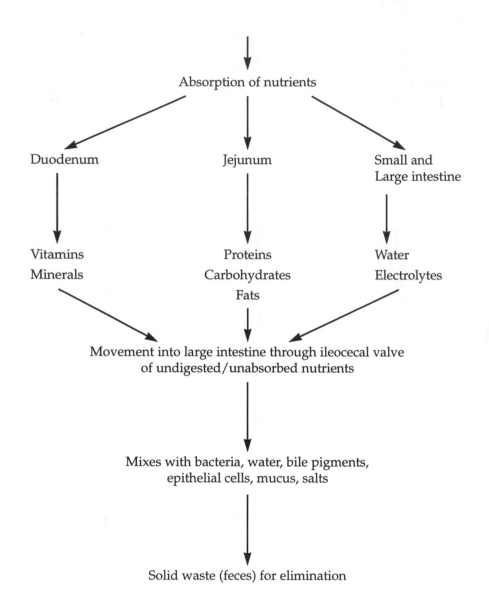

Absorption of nutrients

Duodenum   Jejunum   Small and
Large intestine

Vitamins   Proteins   Water
Minerals   Carbohydrates   Electrolytes
                  Fats

Movement into large intestine through ileocecal valve
of undigested/unabsorbed nutrients

Mixes with bacteria, water, bile pigments,
epithelial cells, mucus, salts

Solid waste (feces) for elimination

CHAPTER II

GASTROINTESTINAL/NUTRITIONAL ASSESSMENTS

A. Age-Related Tips for History Interview
B. History Review
C. Age-Related Tips for Physical
    Examination
D. Physical Assessment
E. Age-Related Tips to Promote Nutrition
F. Nutritional Assessment

Gastrointestinal System History Review

I. Biographical Data:

Name _____

Age ____ Sex ____ Marital Status _____

Children/Family Members _____

Occupation _____

Education_____

Religious Affiliation_____

II. Complaint(s)/Signs and Symptoms:

Anorexia _____ Heartburn_____

Smell_____ Nausea _____

Taste _____ Vomiting _____

Sore Mouth _____ Hematemesis _____

Toothache _____ Flatulence _____

Dentures _____ Bloating/Distention _____

Poor Fitting Dentures _____ Diarrhea _____

Rigid Facial Muscles _____ Constipation_____

Dysphagia _____ Blood in Feces _____

Dyspepsia _____ Rectal Itching_____

Reflux_____ Fecal Incontinence_____

Excessive Belching_____ Other _____

Unintentional Change in Weight_____

III. Past, Present Medical Status:

General Health _____

Gastrointestinal Surgeries_____

Diabetes Mellitus _____ Osteoporosis _____

Heart Disease _____ Cholecystitis_____

Thyroid Dysfunction _____ Hepatic Disease _____

Diverticular Disease _____ Malabsorption Syndrome _____

Hypertension _____ Renal Disease_____

Hiatal Hernia _____ Hemorrhoids _____

Anemia _____ Malnutrition_____

Ulcer Disease _____ Dehydration_____

Intestinal Inflammation/Infection_____

Compromised Skin Integrity _____

Accidents/Falls _____

Other _____

IV. Social Habits:

Alcohol_____ Tobacco Use _____

Caffeinated Beverages_____ Other _____

V. Psychologic Factors:

Anxiety _____ Boredom _____

Stressors_____ Loneliness

Depression_____ Disengagement _____

Grieving_____

Communication Problem _____

Dementia _____ Other _____

VI. Special Considerations:

Special Diet _____

_____

Special Restrictions/Inclusions _____

_____

Food/Drug Allergies_____

Dental Hygiene Pattern_____

Fluid Intake_____

Use of Laxatives, Enemas and Type _____

_____

Prescribed Medications_____

Over-the-Counter Medications and/or Dietary Supplements ___

_____

Exercise/Fatigue Pattern _____

Diagnostic Laboratory and Procedure Studies _____

Other _____

Age-Related Tips for Physical Examination

1. Provide privacy for all aspects of the physical assess-
    ment; use appropriate draping to ensure privacy and
    warmth as the older adult chills easily.

2. Compare normal physiologic aging changes with
    examination results.

3. Allow to empty bladder before examination to prevent
    accidental loss of urine and embarrassment.

4. Place in supine position unless head elevation is needed
    to facilitate breathing and chest expansion; assist to
    change position to sidelying or sitting if needed.

5. Warm hands and stethoscope before touching the skin as
    the older adult has a reduced tolerance to coldness.

6. The abdominal wall is thinner and more relaxed from
    loss of muscle tone; this allows for easier and more
    accurate palpation.

7. The abdomen should be auscultated prior to palpation
    or percussion to prevent changes in bowel sounds; use
    the diaphragm of the stethoscope for auscultation of
    bowel sounds.

8. Examine all four quadrants of the abdomen and count
    the sounds to reveal bowel motility which is often
    reduced in the older adult.

9. The liver edge is more easily palpated because of flattening of the diaphragm.

10. Less pain and abdominal rigidity can be experienced in acute and chronic conditions; abdominal distention is a common distress sign in the older adult.

11. Physical assessment of the gastrointestinal system should begin with the mouth and end with the anus.

Physical Assessment

Area	Method	Normal Findings	Abnormal Findings
Lips	Inspection	Pink color, deeper vertical markings, symmetry during rest or movement	Red, pale, or bluish color; dry, cracked, or chaffed; inflamed fissures at corners; lesions or ulcerations
Oral mucosa	Inspection with tongue blade and penlight	Light or dark pink color; thin, shiny mucosa	White or gray patches; redness, swelling, bleeding, exudate; sore mouth; lesions or ulcerations; dry mouth, halitosis

Area	Method	Normal Findings	Abnormal Findings
Gums	Same as above	Pink color; gums/teeth margin tight; no bleeding or swelling	Red color or pallor; bleeding on pressure; spurs, uneven ridges; lesions or ulcerations; pockets at tooth margins; swelling, pain
Tongue	Same as above	Pink color, moist, shiny, symmetry, smooth and even with fissure	Red color, swelling; lesions, patches; induration, limpness; lateral movement; sublingual varicosities; white exudate
Teeth	Same as above	Yellowish color; firmly set in place; increased exposure of neck of teeth	Tooth loss; loose or broken teeth; wearing down or erosion of teeth; toothache; periodontal disease; partial or full dentures
Pharynx	Same as above with gentle compression to back of tongue	Pink color, smooth; tonsils present or absent; uvula in midline	Redness of tonsils; swelling, exudate, hypertrophy of tonsils; lesions or plaques; uvula in lateral position

Area	Method	Normal Findings	Abnormal Findings
Abdomen	Inspection	Pink color but paler than other parts; smooth and soft; silvery striae, scars from surgeries; umbilicus in center; flat, rounded, concave contour; increased fat deposits; abdominal symmetry; smooth, even movements with breathing; no visible peristalsis or pulsations	Redness, jaundice, cyanosis color; bruises, lesions, rashes; skin taut, shiny; increased abdominal girth, abdominal distention; umbilicus displacement; visible hernia; concavity with wasting; bulges or masses in any area; increased, labored respirations with restricted abdominal movements; marked pulsations and visible peristalsis

Area	Method	Normal Findings	Abnormal Findings
Abdomen	Auscultation with stethoscope diaphragm in all four quadrants	Usually 5-34/minute; sounds vary with gurgles, clicks, soft bubbling every 5-15 seconds	Absence of sound for 5 minutes; infrequent sounds; rapid, high pitched tinkling noises; loud, gurgling noises
	Auscultation with stethoscope bell	Absence of vascular sounds in epigastric, liver, or spleen areas; absence of friction rub over liver or spleen	Bruits (high pitched, soft and swishing over artery); venous hum (low pitched, soft and continuous); friction rub (sounds like sandpaper rubbed together)

Area	Method	Normal Findings	Abnormal Findings
Abdomen	Percussion in all four quadrants	Dull to flat to tympanic depending on air or solid material in bowel; dullness over distended bladder; upper and lower liver borders and liver span and movement within normal parameters; small area of dullness or tympany over spleen	Dullness in any area or a shifting dullness; enlarged liver with lower and upper borders span exceeding normal placement; enlarged spleen with extension of dullness or tympany changing to dullness on inspiration

Area	Method	Normal Findings	Abnormal Findings
Abdomen	Palpation, light and deep	Lax muscle tone; no tenderness except palpation over cecum or sigmoid; smooth feeling with consistent tension; slight inversion or eversion of umbilicus; palpable aorta, feces in colon, palpable femoral pulse; liver border smooth and non-tender if felt on inspiration; spleen nonpalpable; kidneys rarely palpable; small, mobile, soft and smooth inguinal nodes	Rigidity or resistance; deep visceral pain or cutaneous pain; distention; bulging or mass at umbilicus; mobile or fixed masses; enlarged, nodular, irregular, tender liver; tenderness at splenic area; enlarged kidney; tender, enlarged nodes
Bony prominences	Visual inspection	No breaks in skin integrity	Open areas, red areas, excoriation

Physical Assessment

Area	Method	Normal Findings	Abnormal Findings
Rectum	Inspection	Coarse skin with no tenderness	Redness in color; irritation, soreness; lumps, scars; mucosa bulging through anus; tags, hemorrhoids, fissure
	Palpation	Smooth, even pressure on finger, smooth surface of rectal wall	Loss of sphincter muscle tone; fecal impactation
Feces	Inspection; guaiac test	Soft, brown, formed	Black, tarry, chalky; blood, pus, mucus; occult blood; hard, marble-like; loose, watery

Physical Assessment Checklist

Name _____ Male _____ Female _____

General Appearance _____

Anorexia _____ Heartburn_____

Age _____ Ht _____ Wt _____ Frame _____

Body Mass Index (BMI) _____ Waist-Hip ratio _____

Abdominal girth_____

Inspection (Note Abnormalities):

Color, symmetry, texture, lesions, bleeding, odor of:_____

Lips _____ Gums _____ Tongue_____ Teeth_____

Oral mucosa _____ Pharynx_____

Skin color, integrity and lesions, contour and symmetry of:

Abdomen_____ Rectum _____

Feces and characteristics_____

Auscultation (Note Abnormalities):

All quadrants for:

Bowel sounds _____

Blood vessels (aorta, iliac, femoral arteries) for:

Vascular sounds (Bruits)_____

Percussion (Note Abnormalities):

All quadrants for:

Masses _____ Tenderness _____

Liver and Spleen for:

Size _____ Masses_____

Bladder for:

Distention _____

Palpation (Note Abnormalities):

All quadrants for:

Masses _____ Tenderness _____

Liver and Spleen for:

Size _____ Masses _____ Nodules _____

Inguinal Nodes for:

Size _____

Bladder for:

Distention _____

Anus and Rectum for:

Prolapse _____ Fissures _____ Hemorrhoids _____

Tone of Sphincters _____ Masses_____

Changes Related To Nutritional Imbalances:

Eyes _____ Hair _____ Skin _____ Nails _____

Teeth _____ Muscles _____ Skeletal _____

Mucous Membranes _____

Notes:

_____

_____

_____

_____

Age-Related Tips To Promote Nutrition

1. Respect food habits and preferences as they reflect values, beliefs, culture, and emotional status of the older adult which have been developed over many years.

2. Behaviors such as complaining, rejection, or overeating can be evidence of an underlying problem.

3. Be positive and show enthusiasm and encouragement at mealtime.

4. Prepare appropriately prior to meals; provide mouth care, wash hands and face, place in sitting position, insert dentures if applicable. Maintain good oral hygiene.

5. Allow time for eating meal at a slow pace; avoid facial expressions or body language that convey hurriedness.

6. Encourage self-feeding but assist in cutting meat, opening cartons and packages, protecting clothing when needed.

7. Express an attitude that the task is important and worth your time when feeding an older adult.

8. Allow for and accept feelings of frustration, anger, and embarrassment when eating problems exist.

9. Provide adaptive aids for eating when needed to promote self-feeding.

10.   Provide food consistency and texture appropriate for chewing and/or swallowing problems.

11.   Maintain an environment that is clean and orderly, free of odors, and has optimal temperature and ventilation.

12.   Encourage chewing foods well, eating slowly, and taking small bites at one time; explain how this aids digestion.

13.   Encourage intake of a moderate amount of fluids with a meal and explain how this aids digestion and elimination.

14.   Avoid judgmental attitude regarding ethnic food habits, religious restrictions or vegetarian preference.

15.   Be aware of the effect of drugs and emotional status on the nutritional well-being of the older adult (depression, loneliness, anxiety).

16.   Be aware of common physical factors influencing nutritional status such as tooth pain and loss, reduced sense of smell and taste (olfactory and gustatory perception), reduced secretion of saliva, digestive juices, and enzymes, decreased peristalsis, chronic diseases, and physical handicaps.

17.   Communal meals reduce social isolation and loneliness; encourage eating at a table and in a dining room if possible.

18.   Be aware of any dietary modifications related to a medical condition and offer food exchanges according to preferences, physical factors, and appetite.

19.   Provide meals at intervals that will benefit the older adult; 3 meals/day with between meal feedings; 6 meals/day, feedings every 2-4 hours.

20.   Request family to bring seasonings and special foods from home as appropriate.

21.   Avoid interruptions at mealtime for medications or procedures.

22. Note financial resources that determine type and amount of food intake.

23. Offer a variety of foods as monotony causes a loss of interest in eating.

24. Brightly colored meals with garnishes and tablecloth can make meals more appetizing; radio or TV can make mealtime more enjoyable if not overly loud.

25. Assure that food is served at proper temperature.

26. If necessary, adjust timing of medications to enhance oral intake.

NUTRITIONAL ASSESSMENT

Name _____ Age _____ Sex _____ Date _____

Ht ____ Wt____ Frame _____ Recent Loss _____

Recent Gain_____

Minimum, Average, and Maximum Wt in Past Month_____

General State of Health/Appearance _____

Changes in Functional Status (ADL) _____

Chronic Disease(s) _____

Special Dietary Modifications _____

Special Ethnic/Cultural Considerations _____

Food/Drug Allergies_____

Prescribed Drugs _____

Over-the-Counter Drugs
or Other Supplements_____

Food Preferences _____

Preferences in Preparation _____

Food Dislikes/Intolerances _____

_____

Knowledge of Food Guide Pyramid_____

Eating Habits:

Attitude _____ Interest _____ Eat Alone _____

Meals/Day _____ Time of Meals _____ Snacks _____

Amount of Food Consumed/Meal, 24 Hours_____

Calculated Caloric Need/24 Hours _____

Protein _____ Fat _____ Carbohydrate_____

Nutritional Supplement _____ Vitamin/Mineral_____

Amount/Type of Fluid Intake/24 Hours_____

Calculated Fluid Need/24 Hours _____

Bowel Habits:

Frequency _____ Time of Day _____

Characteristics (color, consistency) _____

Constituents (blood, mucus) _____

Eating Problems:

Fatigue _____ Apathy _____

Ability to Feed Self _____

Use of Aids_____ Anorexia _____ Dry Mouth_____

Heartburn _____ Dyspepsia_____

Dentition/Dentures _____ Chewing _____

Swallowing _____

Disabilities:

Paralysis_____ Hand-Arm Coordination _____

Visual Impairment _____ Thirst Impairment_____

Olfactory/Gustatory Impairment _____

Laboratory Test Results:

Protein, Albumin _____

Cholesterol, Low Density Lipoproteins _____

Hematocrit, Hemoglobin, MCV_____

BUN, Creatinine_____

Alternative Feeding/Bowel Elimination Patterns:

Gastrostomy _____ Nasogastric Tube _____

Total Parenteral Nutrition_____

Intravenous Fluids_____ Colostomy _____

24 Hour Food Intake

Meal/Time, Food, Amount of Calories

Breakfast

Time _____

_____

_____

Lunch

Time _____

_____

_____

Dinner

Time _____

_____

_____

Snacks

Time _____

_____

_____

Totals

Total calculated recommended calories _____

Over/Under caloric requirement and amount _____

Number of Servings:

Dairy Products_____ Meats _____ Vegetables _____

Fruits _____

Grains/Bread/Cereals_____

Salt Use _____

Candies/Condiments/Alcohol _____

Food Guide Pyramid Comparison and Needs _____

CHAPTER III

NUTRITIONAL PROBLEMS FOR NURSING CARE PLAN INCLUSION

A. Altered Nutrition: Less Than Body
    Requirements
B. Altered Nutrition: More Than Body
    Requirements
C. Altered Oral Mucous Membrane
D. Altered Tissue Perfusion
    (Gastrointestinal)
E. Bowel Incontinence
F. Constipation
G. Diarrhea
H. Risk for Aspiration
I. Risk for Fluid Volume Deficit
    (Active Loss)
J. Risk for Impaired Skin Integrity
K. Impaired Swallowing
L. Knowledge Deficit
M. Self-Care Deficit, Feeding
N. Sensory/Perceptual Alterations
    (Gustatory, Olfactory)

Altered Nutrition: Less Than Body Requirements

Related Factor:	Inability to ingest food
Defining Characteristics:	Lack of interest in food
	Reduced intake of calories and protein
	Inappropriate use of restricted diets
	Reduced olfactory/gustatory perception
	Administration of multiple medications
	Dysphagia
	Anorexia
	Nausea, vomiting
	Sore mouth
	Poor fitting dentures, toothache
	Difficulty chewing
	Abdominal distention
	Early satiety
	Abdominal pain
	Weight loss (20% or more under ideal)
	Loneliness/depression
Related Factor:	Inability to digest food
Defining Characteristics:	Reduced secretion of digestive juices/enzymes
	Vitamin/mineral deficiency
	Surgeries such as gastric, small or large bowel resection
	Hepatitis, cirrhosis, pancreatitis

	Common bile duct obstruction
	Delayed gastric emptying
Related Factor:	Inability to absorb nutrients
Defining Characteristics:	Diarrhea
	Inadequate absorption surface (surgery of small, large bowel)
	Abnormal bowel motility
	Hyperactive or diminished bowel sounds
	Bacterial overgrowth (antimicrobials)
	Malnutrition
	Vascular insufficiency (reduced circulation to gastrointestinal organs)
Nursing Interventions:	Assess weight at appropriate intervals, food likes and dislikes, cultural and psychological factors, ability to taste, smell, chew and swallow, allergies, medication regimen.
	Assess for conditions that can affect nutrition and cause deficiency, bowel sounds, distention, pain.
	Provide information and rationale for dietary restrictions and inclusions.
	Calculate daily caloric and food group intake and compare to need according to body type, sex, age.
	Monitor trends in weight changes, Hct, Hb, albumin, total protein, electrolyte panel when available.

Provide an environment for meals that is relaxing and pleasant, free from odors/used articles; community dining if possible.

Allow as much independence in food selection and meal times as possible.

Ensure that dentures are in place for meals, oral care given prior to meals if appropriate.

Provide a diet modified for specific needs such as small feedings, supplemental feedings, tube feedings, amounts and consistency, sugar/salt substitutes.

Avoid foods that are gas forming, spicy, contain caffeine; limit fluids prior to meal to prevent early satiety.

Provide ordered special diet associated with medical condition; encourage intake of protein, iron, vitamins and minerals if appropriate.

Provide total parenteral nutrition and care procedures as ordered.

Consult a dietitian for dietary assistance.

Altered Nutrition: More Than Body Requirements

Related Factor:	Excessive intake in relationship to metabolic need
Defining Characteristics:	Weight at least 10% over ideal for height, frame
	Decreased metabolic rate
	Sedentary activity level

Increased intake

Dysfunctional eating pattern (response to internal and external cues other than hunger)

Nursing Interventions:

Assess weight at appropriate intervals, perception of food as a reward or for psychological satisfaction, type of foods preferred, eating patterns, cultural factors that predispose to overweight problems.

Provide information and rationale for dietary changes and changes in lifestyle to promote weight loss. Calculate daily caloric and food group intake and compare to need according to body type, age, sex.

Assist to consider new eating pattern that includes frequency of meals, amount and caloric content of foods, eat only when hungry and not between meals, stop eating when feeling full and avoid overeating.

Allow to select preferred foods within confines of a planned low caloric diet.

Obtain assistance from a dietitian in planning dietary caloric restriction, especially when associated with a medical condition.

Assist in increasing activity level as appropriate. Incorporate other interests in daily routine to decrease focus on food.

Altered Oral Mucous Membrane

Related Factor:	Dehydration
	Ineffective oral hygiene
	Periodontal disease
	Poor fitting dentures
	Decreased salivation, xerostomia
	Thinning and drying of oral epithelium
	Mouth breathing
	Decreased sensation to hot/cold foods
	Malnutrition
	Nasogastric tube
	Medications
Defining Characteristics:	Oral burns, lesions, plaque
	Xerostomia
	Oral pain or discomfort
	Halitosis
	Redness, irritation of mucosa and/or gums
	Bleeding from gums
	Coated tongue
Nursing Interventions:	Assess oral cavity for color, inflammation, lesions, soreness, irritation, condition of teeth, bleeding, dryness, presence of denture, debris, trauma, odor.
	Assess for medication side effects or treatment regimen that can affect oral mucosa.

Assess for oral hygiene pattern and articles used, ability to provide own care.

Provide information and rationale for oral care and treatments.

Provide a routine mouth care plan, assist with tooth-brushing, flossing, mouth rinsing as needed; remove, cleanse, and reinsert dentures as needed.

Apply commercially prepared lubricant to lips and oral cavity as needed.

Offer sugar free chewing gum and hard candies to stimulate saliva for dry mouth if appropriate, increase fluid intake and room humidity if appropriate.

Provide mouth care prior to and following meals.

Use soft brush, foam swabs, gentle brushing or cleansing of teeth and tongue if mucosa is irritated or sore; administer analgesic lozenges if ordered, massage gums if appropriate.

Avoid smoking, foods that are spicy, hot, or irritating to the oral cavity; offer foods that are bland and soft if at risk for oral mucous membrane alteration.

Ensure regular dental check-ups and teeth/denture repair when needed.

Altered Tissue Perfusion (Gastrointestinal)

Related Factor:	Interruption of arterial flow
Defining Characteristics:	Decreased circulation to digestive organs
	Nausea, vomiting
	Abdominal distention, pain
	Abnormal bowel sounds
	Poor nutrition
Nursing Interventions:	Assess abdominal pain (type and location), nausea, vomiting, increasing abdominal girth, bowel sounds, changes in feces characteristics (blood, diarrhea).
	Provide information and rationale for measures that promote circulatory status.
	Provide small amounts of easily ingested and digested foods, fluids as tolerated.
	Provide a restful environment prior to and following meals.
	Insert nasogastric tube and connect to suction as ordered.
	Provide encouragement and support for dietary changes and/or restrictions if long-term.

Bowel Incontinence

Related Factor:	Neuromuscular involvement
	Musculoskeletal involvement
	Anxiety, depression

	Impaired sensory perception/cognitive ability
	Diarrhea, fecal impaction
Defining Characteristics:	Involuntary passage of feces
	Lack of awareness of urge to defecate
	Stained clothing
Nursing Interventions:	Assess frequency and time of incontinence episodes, factors that contribute to incontinence, medical conditions that cause incontinence (spinal cord injury, stroke, intestinal infection or inflammation, others), changes in bowel sounds.
	Assess usual bowel elimination pattern that includes color, amount, consistency and frequency characteristics and compare with bowel incontinence pattern.
	Provide information and rationale for measures to prevent incontinence.
	Establish a schedule for bowel elimination after a meal, use suppository or digital stimulation to empty bowel of feces.
	Provide assistance to bathroom, bedpan at planned intervals or when urge is felt.
	Administer stool softener, bulk forming medications as ordered. Provide cleansing of perianal area and buttocks with pH neutral agent following an incontinence episode to prevent skin irritation.

Provide a diet that includes fiber and bulk, fluid intake increased to 2500 mL/day if allowed.

Provide clean linens when needed, use protective incontinent pad on the bed.

Provide protective pads or underwear to prevent embarrassment caused by soiling of clothing.

Constipation

Related Factor:	Less than adequate bulk/fiber intake
	Less than adequate fluid intake
	Less than adequate physical activity
	Personal habits
	Medications; habitual use of laxatives/enemas
	Neuromuscular impairment
	Musculoskeletal impairment
	Pain on defecation
	Weak abdominal muscles
	Emotional/mental status
Defining Characteristics:	Frequency less than usual pattern
	Hard-formed feces
	Excessive straining during defecation
	Decreased bowel sounds
	Less than usual amount of feces
	Abdominal discomfort, rectal fullness

Flatulence, distention

Palpable mass, fecal impaction

Nursing Interventions:　　　　Assess pattern, factors that affect elimination, feces characteristics; bowel sounds auscultated, distention palpated.

Assess dietary pattern and food inclusion, fluid intake, and amount of activity.

Explain the cause of the constipation and rationale for all nursing care measures.

Provide privacy during elimination and avoid rushing; place tissues and other articles within reach.

Allow time in daily routines to schedule bowel elimination.

Provide immediate assistance to bathroom if urge is felt; avoid behavior that can cause resident to feel that request for assistance is viewed as demanding.

Administer stool softener, bulk forming agents as ordered.

Administer laxative, suppository, enema as ordered if other measures fail to produce bowel elimination.

Provide a balanced diet that includes bulk/fiber foods.

Provide an increased fluid intake of 2-3 L/day, if allowed, that includes citrus/prune juice and warm beverages in the morning before breakfast.

Provide opportunities for exercise and activities; encourage participation.

Perform digital rectal examination and remove fecal impaction if appropriate.

Provide soothing measures for sore, irritated rectal area such as sitz bath or ointment as needed.

Inform of dietary inclusions of high fiber/bulk foods.

Diarrhea

Related Factor:	Stress and anxiety
	Dietary intake
	Medications (antimicrobials, laxatives)
	Malabsorption of bowel
	Bowel infection/inflammation (contaminants, medical condition)
Defining Characteristics:	Abdominal cramping, pain
	Increased frequency
	Loose, liquid feces
	Urgency
	Changes in color and odor of feces
	Increased motility/bowel sounds
	Positive culture for toxins, causative organism
	Temperature elevation

Nursing Interventions:

Assess onset, frequency, amount, and characteristics of diarrheal output; dietary, medication, or gastrointestinal condition (bacterial, inflammatory) associated with diarrhea, weight loss, changes in bowel sounds.

Assess for associated signs and symptoms such as fever, abdominal pain/cramping, dehydration, stress.

Explain the cause of diarrhea and rationale for care and treatments.

Provide liquid diet or NPO to rest the tract for a limited time; IV to replace fluids if loss is severe.

Provide dietary modification that includes a high protein, high calorie, low fiber content and excludes milk, raw fruits and vegetables, spicy and gas-forming foods.

Increase fluid intake to 2,500 mL/day if allowed, limit caffeine-containing beverages and include bouillon, juices, and commercially prepared electrolyte solutions (Gatorade).

Gradually resume normal dietary and fluid intake as diarrhea subsides; offer yogurt to restore bowel flora.

Administer antidiarrheal as ordered.

Monitor I&O, measure diarrheal output.

Cleanse anal area with pH neutral agent following each elimination and pat dry; apply protective ointment if needed to prevent excoriation caused by frequent diarrheal bowel elimination.

Provide protective pad or underwear if needed to prevent embarrassment.

Risk for Aspiration

Related Factor:	Decreased gag reflex
	Decreased peristalsis activity/gastrointestinal motility
	Relaxation of lower esophageal sphincter
	Reduced level of consciousness
	Gastrointestinal feeding tube
	Increased gastric residual
	Delayed gastric emptying
	Impaired swallowing
Defining Characteristics:	Choking, coughing
	Vomiting, nausea
	Dysphagia
	Aspiration pneumonia
Nursing Interventions:	Assess level of consciousness, cognitive abilities, gag/swallowing reflex impairment, ability to clear airways, presence of respiratory secretions or vomiting, change in breath sounds.
	Provide information and rationale for food and eating modifications to prevent aspiration.

Provide semi-solid foods, feed slowly in small pieces and amounts, and allow time to chew foods; avoid pureed or blenderized foods and taking fluids with solid foods when swallowing.

Ensure that daily requirement for calories and fluids are ingested.

Place in upright position for eating and drinking, avoid using a straw to drink fluids.

Provide mouth care following eating to ensure that all food is removed from oral cavity. If gastric tube is in place, check placement and for residual prior to feedings.

Administer medications in liquid or crushed tablet form.

Confer with speech therapist as indicated for swallowing, evaluation, safe swallow techniques.

Maintain suctioning equipment at the bedside to remove food, fluids, secretions from trachea as needed.

Obtain pulmonary secretions for culture studies if pneumonia is suspected (fever, chills, chest pain).

Remain and observe during meals if tendency to choke on food or swallowing impairment is present.

Risk for Fluid Volume Deficit (Active Loss)

Related Factor:

Extremes in age

Excessive losses via diarrhea, vomiting, other normal routes

Loss of fluids via indwelling tubes, other abnormal routes

Inability to secure fluids (immobility)

Medication (diuretic)

Altered intake

Impaired thirst sensation

Defining Characteristics: Decreased urine output (concentrated)

Fluid output greater than intake

Decreased fluid intake

Dehydration

Electrolyte imbalance (Na, K)

Thirst, dry skin and mucous membranes, decreased skin turgor

Weight loss

Weakness

Temperature elevation

Change in mentation

Nursing Interventions: Assess for signs and symptoms of dehydration or electrolyte imbalance, source of fluid loss (bleeding, vomiting, diarrhea, respirations, perspiration, drainage), medical conditions associated with fluid deficit (bowel inflammatory disease, abdominal malignancy).

Assess vital signs for decreased blood pressure, increased pulse, decreased pulse volume and pressure, capillary refill, urine specific gravity.

Impaired Swallowing

Related Factor:	Neuromuscular impairment
	Fatigue
	Limited awareness
Defining Characteristics:	Absent gag reflex
	Inability to chew food
	Rigidity of facial muscles
	Coughing/choking
	Stasis of food in oral cavity
Nursing Interventions:	Assess ability to swallow and use muscles for chewing.
	Explain and provide rationale for care and promotion of swallowing measures.
	Monitor tongue, lips, and facial muscle movements, weight gain or loss.
	Provide oral care prior to and following meals to promote appetite and remove food particles left in mouth.
	Provide an environment that is pleasant and avoids distractions during meals.
	Feed or assist to eat in an upright position; advise to eat one food at a time in small amounts and allow time to eat and swallow slowly; advise to place head forward to enhance swallowing.

Provide semi-solid foods, thick or slushy fluids that are more easily manipulated in the mouth and advise to place food at the back of the mouth or unaffected side if appropriate. Avoid use of straws and drinking fluids to assist in swallowing food. Administer medications in liquid or crushed form if possible.

Confer with speech therapist to evaluate swallow and determine safe swallow techniques.

Maintain suction supplies and equipment at the bedside to prevent possible aspiration.

Knowledge Deficit

Related Factor:	Lack of recall
	Cognitive limitation
	Lack of interest in learning
	Requests no information
Defining Characteristics:	Communication impairment
	Intellectual impairment
	Agitation, apathy
	Inability to perform activities or manage own medical regimen
Nursing Interventions:	Assess knowledge of physical/psychosocial implications of disease, medical regimen, expectations related to own behavior, ability and/or readiness to learn, willingness to participate in own care.

Assess factors to be considered in learning such as educational level, age, cultural aspects/language barrier, sensory/cognitive deficits.

Provide rationale for information given to promote understanding.

Prioritize identified content to be learned and limit sessions to prevent fatigue or disinterest.

Provide an environment that is comfortable, free from distractions.

Provide information regarding existing medical conditions and risk for other disorders, need for fluid/nutritional intake, sleep and rest, exercise, bowel/bladder elimination, other areas related to gastrointestinal system.

Utilize teaching aids such as videotapes, models, charts, pictures, others if appropriate.

Provide information in writing if and when appropriate.

Provide opportunity for group teaching if desired.

Self-Care Deficit, Feeding

Related Factor: Neuromuscular/musculoskeletal impairment

Depression

Disorientation

Cognitive impairment

Pain or discomfort

Defining Characteristics:	Inability to feed self or manipulate utensils
	Paralysis
	Reduced state of consciousness
	Weakness, fatigue
	Unable to use assistive aid
	Unable to lift glass/food to mouth
	Unable to cut meat, butter bread
Nursing Interventions:	Explain rationale for progressive self-feeding, use of assistive aids as appropriate.
	Place in a semi-Fowler's or upright position as tolerated to prepare for complete or assistive feeding; transport to dining room if possible.
	Arrange items on the tray and place within reach, open packaged items, cut meat, break egg, butter bread, place napkin on chest, and assist as needed depending on abilities.
	Provide drinking straw, padded utensil handles, large handled cups.
	Perform complete feeding by positioning of resident and sitting down while feeding, preparing the tray; provide an explanation of the food and fluids on the tray and request preferences; instruct to indicate when finished with meal.
	Provide small amounts of food and allow time to chew and swallow to prevent choking, feed slowly to prevent fatigue. Allow family member to feed if desired.

Sensory/Perceptual Alterations (Gustatory, Olfactory)

Related Factor:	Aging
	Chronic illness
	Altered status of sense organs (olfactory/gustatory)
	Sleep deprivation
	Medications
Defining Characteristics:	Change in taste and smell affecting eating
	Disorientation
	Apathy, anxiety
	Change in behavior pattern
Nursing Interventions:	Assess for complaints involving changes in the way food tastes; affect of odors and changes in taste on appetite and eating.
	Provide an odor free, well-ventilated dining environment.
	Allow expression of frustration, deprivation and include in food selection for meal planning.
	Provide foods that are requested, add spices and other condiments that accentuate taste.
	Assure adequate oral hygiene before and after meals.

CHAPTER IV

ESSENTIAL NUTRIENTS AND FUNCTIONS

Basic Food Groups

Food Group	Servings Required/Day	Nutrients Supplied
Bread/Cereals/ Grains/Pasta/Rice	6-11 servings	Complex carbohydrate, thiamin, niacin, vitamins B_6, E, magnesium, iron, zinc, folic acid
Fruits/Vegetables	5-9 servings that include 1 citrus fruit and 1 green or yellow vegetable	Carbohydrates, thiamin, niacin, vitamins A, C, B_6, E, phosphorus, potassium, magnesium, calcium, iron, fiber, folic acid
Meat/Fish/Eggs/ Legumes/Nuts	2-3 servings	Protein, thiamin, niacin, riboflavin, vitamins A, E, iron, iodine, phosphorus, magnesium, zinc
Dairy Products	2-3 servings	Protein, vitamins A, D, B_6, B_{12}, calcium, phosphorus, zinc, magnesium
Supplementary Foods/Condiments	No specific requirements, but should be considered in meal planning	Alcohol, chocolate, caffeinated beverages, jam/jelly, candy, syrup, pastry, cookies, potato chips, snack foods, mayonnaise, butter, olives, margarine, seasonings, catsup, pickles, mustard, spices

FOOD PYRAMID

The food pyramid is a model to serve as a guide to choose foods and the number of servings to eat daily. The three lower levels should be included in a diet to supply all the nutrients, vitamins and minerals needed for good health. The least number of servings from each food group daily should supply the amount of calories needed by the older adult but these must be modified according to sex, weight, height, and general health needs. The fourth level contains the fats and sweets group which may or may not be included in the other food groups. If more food is needed, it should be selected from the lower three groups, not the foods included in the top of the pyramid. The pyramid developed by the U.S. Department of Agriculture/U.S. Department of Health and Human Services is portrayed below: (Fig. 4.1)

Food Guide Pyramid
A Guide to Daily Food Choices

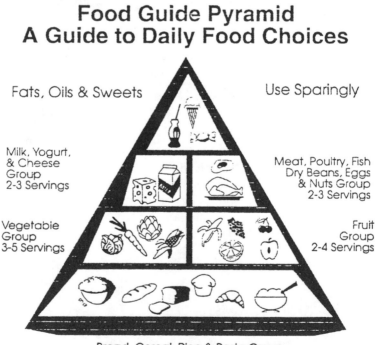

Fats, Oils & Sweets — Use Sparingly

Milk, Yogurt, & Cheese Group 2-3 Servings

Meat, Poultry, Fish Dry Beans, Eggs & Nuts Group 2-3 Servings

Vegetable Group 3-5 Servings

Fruit Group 2-4 Servings

Bread, Cereal, Rice & Pasta Group 6-11 Servings

Recommended Daily Dietary Allowance (Age 51+)*

The recommended dietary allowance (RDA) is considered to be influenced by the aging process in the older adult, and developed from those available for younger adults. Adjustments have been made based on the reduction in physiologic function, changes in body composition, and metabolic adaptation in adults over 51 years of age. Chronic disease and medication regimens, more common in the older adult, also influence nutritional requirements. The following information offers a range of suggested food intakes to (1) present desired amounts to use in dietary planning, (2) prevent conditions caused by deficiency, and (3) provide safe amounts to prevent toxic conditions. Because of individual differences however, specific recommendations should be adjusted to health status and physical activity, as well as essential nutritional intake, to promote healthy successful aging.

Dietary Reference Intake (DRI)

The Institute of Medicine is currently involved in developing Dietary Reference Intakes which will update and expand the RDA's. These new values reflect the latest understanding about nutrient requirements based on optimal health in individuals and groups.

Those nutrients where DRI is listed are noted by an asterisk (*).

Substance	Male: Wt. 170 lb/77 kg Ht. 68 in/173 cm	Female: Wt. 143 lb/65 kg Ht. 63 in/160 cm
Food Nutrients		
Protein	63 g or 10% of calories/day	50 g or 10% of calories/day
Carbohydrate	55-60% of total calories/day	
Fat	30% of total calories/day	
Calories	2,300 kcal/day or 30 kcal/kg	1,900 kcal/day or 30 kcal/day

Substance	Male: Wt. 170 lb/77 kg Ht. 68 in/173 cm	Female: Wt. 143 lb/65 kg Ht. 63 in/160 cm
Vitamins and Minerals		
Vit. A	1,000 µg	800 µg
Vit. B_1 (Thiamin)	1.2 mg	1.0 mg
Vit. B_2 (Riboflavin)	1.4 mg	1.2 mg
Vit. B_6 (Pyridoxine)	2.0 mg	1.6 mg
Vit. B_3 (Niacin)	15 mg	13 mg
Vit. B_{12} (Cyanocobalamin)	2.0 µg	2.0 µg
Vit. C (Ascorbic Acid)	60 mg	60 mg
Vit. D (Calciferol)*	25 µg	25 µg
Vit. E (Tocopherol)	10 mg	8 mg
Vit. K	80 µg	65 µg
Folate	200 µg	180 µg
Biotin	30-100 µg	30-100 µg
Pantothenic Acid	4.0-7.0 mg	4.0-7.0 mg
Calcium*	1200 mg	1200 mg
Chloride	750 mg	750 mg
Potassium	2,000 mg	2,000 mg
Sodium	500 mg	500 mg
Phosphorus*	700 mg	700 mg
Magnesium*	420 mg	320 mg
Manganese	2.0-5.0 mg	2.0-5.0 mg
Selenium	70 µg	55 µg
Copper	1.5-3.0 mg	1.5-3.0 mg
Fluoride*	3.8 mg	3.1 mg
Chromium	500-200 µg	50-200 µg
Molybdenum	75-250 µg	75-250 µg
Iron	10 mg	10 mg
Zinc	15 mg	12 mg
Iodine	150 µg	150 µg

Prepublication copy. "Dietary Reference Intakes: 1: Calcium, Magnesium, Phosphorus, Vitamin D and Flouride." Standing Committee on Scientific Evaluation of Dietary Reference Intakes, Institute of Medicine. National Academy Press: 1998.

Food Nutrients

The three main categories of foods are proteins, carbohydrates, and fats. Proteins, the building blocks, are classified as essential or nonessential amino acids. Essential amino acids cannot be synthesized and must come from foods; nonessential amino acids are those that can be synthesized by the body to meet requirements. Carbohydrates, the provider of the most efficient form of energy, are classified into monosaccharides, disaccharides, and polysaccharides. Fats, the body's most concentrated source of energy, include fatty acids, triglycerides, cholesterol, and phospholipids.

Proteins

RDA	10% of total calories/day or 63 g/day for males and 50 g/day for females
Principle sources	Complete protein: milk and milk products except butter, meat, fish, poultry, eggs, seafoods
	Incomplete protein: legumes, nuts, cereals, rice, pasta, breads; can be consumed in combination with a complete protein, e.g., peanut butter and bread sandwich
Function in body	Replace body nitrogen losses and maintain body tissues
	Formation of hormones, enzymes, antibodies
	Regulate fluid balance of cells and maintain acid-base balance (blood neutrality)
Deficiency	Wasting of muscle tissue, weight loss, delayed healing of wounds and fractures, infection, edema
Persons at risk	Older adults: acute or chronic illness, malnutrition, vegetarianism, immobility

Comments	1 g protein = 4 kcal
	Infection, chronic disease, emotional stress, all of which are common in older adults, increase protein requirements
	Loss of body protein is a function of aging and results in a reduction of body muscle mass

Carbohydrates

RDA	50-55% of total calories/day or 150-300 g/day
Principle sources	Complex carbohydrate: cereal grains, whole grains, fruit, vegetables, sugar, honey
	Other carbohydrate: sugar and sweets, foods high in sucrose
Function in body	First substances to be used to produce energy
	Regulate body processes by its content in hormones, enzymes, nervous tissue, RNA, DNA
	Indigestible portions promote bowel function
Deficiency	Metabolism of protein and fat for energy, breakdown of body tissues
Persons at risk	Diabetes mellitus
Comments	1 g carbohydrate = 4 kcal
	Alcohol yield: 1 g = 7 kcal
	Overconsumption of sugars contributes to obesity, dental disease, and disorders of lipid metabolism

Excess carbohydrate is stored as glycogen and body fat

Reduction diets that substitute protein for carbohydrate can be dangerous to the older adult's renal system and are inappropriate

Fats

RDA	No more than 30% of total calories/day with <10% of saturated fat, 10-15% of monounsaturated fat, 10% of polyunsaturated fat, and 300 mg/day cholesterol
Principle sources	Whole milk and milk products, meat, fish, poultry, oils, margarine, olives, avocados, nuts, seeds
Function in body	Concentrated source of energy in form of fatty acids
	Insulate, cushion
	Transport and support absorption of fat soluble vitamins
Deficiency	Dermatitis, disturbance in fat metabolism
Excess	Obesity, atherosclerosis
Persons at risk	Arterial insufficiency, hypertension, coronary artery disease, gallbladder or liver disease
Comments	1 g fat = 9 kcal
	Common terminology regarding fats include saturated, polyunsaturated, and cholesterol, high or low density lipids

Dietary fat intake can be reduced/modified by using low fat dairy products, reducing intake of meats that are high in saturated fats, and increasing intake of fish, poultry, and vegetables, all of which substitute polyunsaturated fats for saturated fats

Vitamins

Vitamins are organic compounds derived from the diet. Very small quantities are needed to promote growth and maintain health and life. The following provides necessary information about the major vitamins (fat and water soluble) in order to understand their functions, sources, adverse effects of deficiencies and toxicities, and the daily requirements for the older adult. The intake of specific vitamins in the older adult is related to the development of chronic diseases such as cancer, coronary heart disease, cataracts, osteoporosis, and physiologic processes such as immune function, neural function, tissue repair, and red blood cell formation.

Vitamin A (Fat Soluble)

RDA	5,000 IU or 1,000 µg/day for males and 4,000 IU or 800 µg/day for females
Principle sources	Preformed vitamin A: egg yolk, liver, lamb, milk, butter, cheese, margarine
	Precursor carotenoids: yellow-orange pigment foods such as apricots, cantaloupe, peaches, carrots, sweet potatoes, yellow squash, and green vegetables such as broccoli, spinach
Function in body	Vision at night
	Maintain epithelial tissues and mucous membranes and secretions

	Synthesis of steroid hormone
	Formation of bone and cartilage growth
	Repair of cells, resistance of infection
	Dental development
	Spermatogenesis
Storage in body	Liver
Overdose symptoms	Greater than 50,000 IU/day for 2-3 weeks: lethargy, anorexia, drying and desquamation of skin, headache, sweating, bone pain, jaundice, alopecia, photophobia, hepatomegaly, splenomegaly
Deficiency symptoms	Night blindness, spots, xerophthalmia, keratinization of epithelial tissue, hyperkeratosis
Persons at risk	Older adult: diabetes mellitus, hyperthyroidism, alcoholism, smokers
Antagonists	Air pollution, strong light, mineral oil, increased protein intake
Synergists	Vitamins C, D, E
Comments	Absorbed in the small intestine
	Liver vitamin stores are depleted by weight loss, infection, and chronic disease states
	Carotine is the precursor to vitamin A, is fat soluble and insoluble in water; supplements of beta-carotene can affect the immune system in older adults

Vitamin D-Calciferol (Fat Soluble)

DRI	1000 IU or 25 µg/day for males and females (in absence of sunlight)
Principle sources	Vitamin D fortified milk, sunlight, liver oils, margarine, lard, egg yolks, butter, shrimp, salmon, tuna
Function in body	Growth and repair of bone
	Regulate and maintain calcium and phosphorus balance and absorption in the intestine
Storage in body	Liver and skin
Overdose symptoms	Calcification of skin, blood vessels, kidneys, and other soft tissue, anorexia, diarrhea, polyuria, muscle weakness, kidney stones
Deficiency symptoms	Osteomalacia, hypothyroidism, tetany, osteoporosis, tooth decay, decreased muscle tone
Persons at risk	Older adults deprived of sunlight; non-milk drinkers
Antagonists	Cortisone, anticonvulsants
Synergists	Vitamins A, B_1, B_3, C, and calcium
Comments	Mild or serious permanent bone deformities
	Older adults synthesize less cholecalciferol (D_3) because of skin changes
	Older adults have less exposure to sunlight, especially if debilitated and limited in physical activity
	Many older adults do not drink milk

Vitamin E-Tocopherol (Fat Soluble)

RDA	10 mg/day for males and 8 mg/day for females
Principle sources	Vegetable oil, margarine, peanuts, whole grains, chocolate, yeast, cabbage, broccoli, asparagus, spinach
Function in body	Metabolism of fats
	Antioxidant
	Maintain cell membrane integrity
	Prevent premature aging
	Protect against lung damage from pollutants and smoking
	Aid in stress response of body
Storage in body	Highest concentration in liver, pituitary gland, testes, and adrenal glands
Overdose symptoms	Possible increase in blood pressure, interference with clotting function
Deficiency symptoms	Anemia, degeneration of reproductive tissue and muscle, liver necrosis
Antagonists	Rancid fats and oils, iron if taken at same time, mineral oil, thyroid hormone
Synergists	Vitamins A, B complex, C, and cortisone, testosterone
Comments	Avoid taking with iron preparation
	It is believed that vitamin E can improve the immune response and offers cardiac protection

Vitamin K (Fat Soluble)

RDA	80 µg for males and 65 µg for females reported, but manufactured in the intestine daily
Principle sources	Mainly green vegetables; also liver, kidney, beef, pork, cauliflower
Function in body	Synthesis of prothrombin and other blood clotting factors by the liver
Storage in body	Liver, produced daily by intestinal flora
Overdose symptoms	Vomiting, possible thrombosis, porphyrinuria
Deficiency symptoms	Hypoprothrombinemia, hemorrhage or tendency to bleed easily
Persons at risk	Chronic diarrhea or disorders that interfere with intestinal absorption
Antagonists	Anticoagulants, penicillin, tetracycline, sulfonamides, aspirin, mineral oil
Synergists	Vitamins A, C, E
Comments	Requires the presence of bile for absorption in the upper part of the small intestine

Vitamin B₁-Thiamin (Water Soluble)

RDA	1.2 mg/day for males and 1.0 mg/day for females
Principle sources	Yeast, wheat germ, whole grains, enriched bread, nuts, pork, liver, plums, prunes, raisins, asparagus, corn, peas, rice, beans, potatoes

Function in the body	Metabolism of carbohydrate
	Synthesis of acetylcholine for health of nerve fibers and neurons
	Aid in digestion
Storage in body	Small amount concentrated in muscles, brain, kidneys, liver, and heart
Overdose symptoms	Greater than 6,000 mg/day: edema, tremors, tachycardia, fatty liver, sweating, hypotension
Deficiency symptoms	Nerve degeneration, fatigue, anorexia, weight loss, muscular atrophy, mental disturbances (depression)
Persons at risk	Older adult; alcoholism, postsurgical status, cardiac conditions, long-term hemodialysis, chronic febrile conditions
Antagonists	Raw fish, tea, coffee, emotional stress, alcohol, antibiotics, nitrates, baking soda
Synergists	Vitamins B_2, B_3, B_6, B_{12}, C, D, pantothenic acid
Comments	Absorbed in the duodenum and jejunum, but can be impaired with use of alcohol
	Folic acid is required for absorption
	Great amount lost in preparation of foods in water

Vitamin B$_2$-Riboflavin (Water Soluble)

RDA	1.4 mg/day for males and 1.2 mg/day for females
Principle sources	Milk, meat, fish, poultry, whole grains, liver, heart, kidney, eggs, avocados, beans, asparagus, broccoli, corn, peas, spinach
Function in body	Maintain epithelium, eye, mucous membranes
	Part of respiratory enzymes
	Component of oxidases that oxidize fatty acids and amino acids
Storage in body	Mainly in the liver and kidneys, intakes above daily needs are excreted by the kidneys
Overdose symptoms	Essentially nontoxic
Deficiency symptoms	Angular stomatitis, glossitis, photophobia, conjunctivitis, seborrheic dermatitis, cracks at mouth corners, photophobic
Persons at risk	Older adult: chronic alcoholism, severe gastrointestinal diseases that interfere with absorption, achlorhydria, hyperthyroidism
Antagonists	Antibiotics
Synergists	Vitamins A, B$_3$, E
Comments	Absorbed rapidly in the duodenum
	Easily destroyed by alkali as in pasteurized milk, use of baking soda to preserve the green color in vegetables or in preparation of meat by baking

Vitamin B₃-Niacin, Nicotinic Acid, Nicotinamide, Niacinamide (Water Soluble)

RDA	15 mg/day for males and 13 mg/day for females
Principle sources	Liver, poultry, fish, yeast, peanuts, enriched grain products, most vegetables
Function in body	Metabolism of proteins, carbohydrates, and fats, pigment metabolism
	Synthesis of fatty acids and cholesterol
	Electron transport in cellular respiratory reactions
Storage in body	Heart, liver, and muscles (limited) with any excess excreted by the kidneys
Overdose symptoms	3,000 mg/day or more: flushing, burning and itching skin, fatty liver, arrhythmias, gastrointestinal problems
Deficiency symptoms	Pellagra with dermatitis, diarrhea, dementia, anorexia, weakness
Persons at risk	Alcoholism, hyperthyroidism, gastrointestinal conditions, diabetes mellitus
Antagonists	Antibiotics, emotional and physical stress
Synergists	Vitamins A, B₁, B₂, B₆, B₁₂, C, D
Comments	Absorbed in the small intestine
	Niacin is used therapeutically to control serum cholesterol levels

Vitamin B₆-Pyridoxine, Pyridoxal, Pyridoxamine (Water Soluble)

RDA	2.0 mg/day for males and 1.6 mg/day for females
Principle sources	Fish, poultry, meats, milk, wheat germ, brown rice, potatoes, peanuts, molasses, walnuts, soybeans, lima beans, yeast, vegetables
Function in body	Metabolism of proteins, carbohydrates, fats
	Maintain immune function and synthesis of neurotransmitters
	Formation of erythrocytes
Storage in body	Leukocytes, nerve tissue, and liver with excess excreted by kidneys as pyridoxic acid
Overdose symptoms	More than 1,000 mg/day: sensory neuropathy
Deficiency symptoms	Seborrheic dermatitis, glossitis, angular stomatitis, peripheral neuropathy, anemia
Persons at risk	Chronic alcoholism, malabsorption syndromes
Antagonists	Isonicotine hydrazine, antihypertensives, levodopa, cortisone, penicillamine
Synergists	Vitamins B_1, B_2, B_3, C, magnesium
Comments	Absorption not known but is found in the extracellular fluid
	Coenzyme in metabolism of protein and amino acids
	Decline in immune function and decreased number of lymphocytes can result from deficiency in the older adult

Serious diseases such as diabetes, heart or renal conditions can cause deficiency in spite of adequate dietary intake

Included in RDA in 1968

Folic Acid, Folate

RDA	200 ug/day for males and 180 ug/day for females
	Experts now recommend 400 ug/day
Principle sources	Cold cereal, dry beans, broccoli, asparagus, spinach, orange juice, fortified flour products
Function in body	Synthesis of choline, DNA, RNA and amino acids
	Coenzyme in purine, pyrimidine metabolism, homocysteine metabolism
Storage in body	Mostly in liver and excreted in urine and feces
Overdose symptoms	No toxicity reported
Deficiency symptoms	Pernicious anemia, macrocytic anemia, sprue, glossitis, leukopenia, thrombocytopenia
Persons at risk	Alcoholism, leukemia, intestinal disorders, older adult, Hodgkin's disease
Antagonists	Antimalarials, anticonvulsants, alcohol, sulfonamides, methotrexate
Synergists	B complex vitamins, vitamin C, and hormones testosterone and estradiol

Comments	Absorption in proximal small intestine in an acidic environment
	Deficiency is usually concurrent with vitamin C deficiency
	Synthesis by upper small intestinal flora
	Folic acid exerts protective effect on cardiac tissue

Vitamin B_{12}-Cobalamin, Cyanocobalamin (Water Soluble)

RDA	2.0 µg/day for males and females
Principle sources	Lamb and beef kidney; lamb, beef, calf and pork liver; beef brain, egg yolk, clams, oysters, sardines, herring, salmon
Function in body	Required by all cells, especially bone marrow, nervous system, and gastrointestinal tract
	Essential to red blood cell formation
	Regulate maturation of erythrocytes
Storage in body	Liver for 3-5 years
Overdose symptoms	No known toxic effects
Deficiency symptoms	Pernicious anemia (pallor, weight loss, glossitis, sprue, anorexia)
	Moodiness, memory loss
Persons at risk	Some vegetarians, surgical removal of stomach, lack of intrinsic factor that prevents absorption of B_{12}
Antagonists	Aspirin, codeine, neomycin
Synergists	Vitamins A, B_1, C, E, folic acid, biotin, pantothenic acid

Comments	Cobalamin containing enzymes involved in the transfer of carbon units
	Defect in absorption caused by lack of intrinsic factor production by chief cells in the stomach
	Synthesized by intestinal flora

Vitamin C-Ascorbic Acid (Water Soluble)

RDA	60 mg/day for males and females
Principle sources	Fresh, frozen, or raw fruits and vegetables, especially citrus fruits
Function in body	Convert folic acid to an active form
	Wound healing; aids in fighting infection, injury and stress
	Maintain body structure and metabolism of some amino acids
	Synthesis of steroids from cholesterol
	Reduction of ferric iron to ferrous iron for absorption
	Maintain capillaries and acts as an antioxidant
Storage in body	Adrenal glands, kidneys, spleen, liver, pancreas, pituitary gland; after tissues are saturated the excess is excreted
Overdose symptoms	Edema, tremors, impaired WBC activity, tachycardia, fatty liver; possible kidney stones and damage to pancreas; excessive iron absorption

Deficiency symptoms	Scurvy, aching joints and muscles, poor wound healing, muscular weakness, anorexia, ecchymoses, bleeding gums, loose teeth, petechiae
Persons at risk	Wounds or surgical incisions, high level of stress, older male adults, smokers
Antagonists	Smoking, pollution, alcohol, aspirin, diuretics, prednisone, antidepressants, anticoagulants, indomethacin
Synergists	B complex vitamins, vitamins A, K, E, and the hormone testosterone
Comments	Absorbed from the gastrointestinal tract
	Easily destroyed by oxidation (prolonged cooking, exposure to iron, oxygen, copper, light, and alkali)
	Slicing food releases oxidative enzymes from surfaces
	Thought to assist in prevention of cataracts and atherosclerosis

Biotin-B Complex

RDA	30-100 µg/day for males and females
Principle sources	Liver, yeast, meats, seafoods, nuts, corn, soybeans, eggs, mushrooms, chocolate
Function in body	Metabolism of carbohydrate, fat, and protein
	Maintain skin, hair, nerves, and bone marrow

Storage in body	Small amounts in liver, kidneys, brain, and adrenals with excretion in urine and feces
Overdose symptoms	Nontoxic in humans
Deficiency symptoms	Muscle pain, anorexia, nausea, vomiting, glossitis, scaly skin, depression
Persons at risk	Alcoholism
Antagonists	Raw egg whites, antibiotics, sulfonamides
Synergists	B complex vitamins, vitamins A, D
Comments	Synthesized by intestinal flora

Pantothenic Acid-B Complex

RDA	4.0-7.0 mg/day for males and females
Principle sources	Liver, kidney, eggs, yeast, wheat germ, dried peas, peanuts, meats, cheese, clams, herring, salmon, mackerel, oats, soybeans, rice, and widely distributed in foods
Function in body	Cellular metabolism of proteins, carbohydrates and fats
	Synthesis of fatty acids, steroids, cholesterol, acetylcholine, porphyrin
Storage in body	Heart, liver, brain, kidneys, and adrenal glands
Overdose symptoms	No known toxicity in humans
Deficiency symptoms	Not usual but can be induced: fatigue, malaise, numbness, muscle cramps, burning of feet, insomnia, nausea, abdominal cramping, indigestion, susceptibility to infection, impaired muscular coordination

Persons at risk	Wounds, physical or emotional stress
Antagonists	Insecticides
Synergists	B complex vitamins, vitamins A, C, E, calcium
Comments	Stable under ordinary cooking procedures

Minerals

Minerals are substances in the human body involved in hormonal activity, oxygen transport, maintenance of fluid and electrolyte balance, osmotic pressure, muscle contraction, the response of nerves to stimuli, and many other functions necessary for health and life. Minerals are present in large and trace amounts (trace elements). Specific minerals can be involved in degenerative and functional changes related to aging in the older adult.

Calcium (Ca)

DRI	1200 mg/day for males and females
Principle sources	Milk and dairy products, spinach, mustard, collard, and turnip greens, shrimp, clams, oysters, salmon, citrus juices fortified with Ca
Function in body	Catalyst for conversion of prothrombin into thrombin
	Muscle contraction
	Transmission of nerve impulses
	Activation of enzymes
	Control of integrity of cement substances and cell membranes

Storage in body	Body contains 1,200-1,250 g of Ca with 99% in bones and teeth and 1% in extracellular fluids and cell membranes
	Most eliminated in the feces with a small amount in urine and sweat
Overdose symptoms	Hypercalcemia, cardiac arrhythmias, lethargy, weakness, muscle flaccidity, headache, anorexia, nausea, vomiting
Deficiency symptoms	Tetany with muscular twitching, tremors, paresthesia, spasmodic contractions, osteoporosis with spontaneous fractures
Persons at risk	Older adult, parathyroid and calcitonin secretion dysfunction, vitamin D deficiency, malabsorption syndromes
Antagonists	High phosphorus diet
Synergists	Vitamin D, high protein diet, lactose
Comments	Absorbed in the duodenum as Ca salts; more soluble in an acid medium
	30% of dietary Ca is absorbed by the adult, but absorption decreases with age
	Increase motility and achlorhydria; decrease absorption
	Gradual loss of bone Ca associated with aging
	Ca loss from the bones accelerate in the first 5 years of postmenopause, then tapers off

Phosphorus (P)

DRI	700 mg/day for males and females
Principle sources	Milk and milk products, lean meats, poultry, fish, grain products; found in most foods
Function in body	Transport fat in the blood
	Transport of substances in and out of cells
	Glucose absorption in the intestine and uptake by cells and reabsorption by renal tubules
	Storage and release of energy (ATP, ADP)
	Activate B vitamins
Storage in body	80-90% in bones and teeth with the remainder in all cells in the form of phosphate ion (PO_4) with elimination in urine and feces
Overdose symptoms	Renal disease, hypoparathyroidism, hypocalcemia with tetany (muscular twitching, tremors, paresthesia), hyperphosphatemia, poor urinary output
Deficiency symptoms	Malabsorption (sprue or celiac disease), bone disease (osteomalacia), muscle weakness, hypophosphatemia, malnutrition, hypercalcemia
Persons at risk	Kidney disease, parathyroid dysfunction
Antagonists	Iron, calcium, aluminum
Synergists	B vitamins, vitamin D, glucose
Comments	Absorption in the intestines after breakdown by enzymes (phosphatases)

Dietary phosphorus should equal calcium intake

Prolonged use of antacids containing aluminum hydroxide can cause phosphorus deficiency by preventing its absorption

Magnesium (Mg)

DRI	420 mg/day for males and 320 mg/day for females
Principle sources	Whole grains, legumes, green leafy vegetables, seafoods, nuts, cocoa, bananas
Function in body	Catalyst for biological reactions
	Transmission of nerve impulses
	Active transport across cell membranes
	Muscle contractions
	Transfer ATP to a phosphate acceptor
Storage in body	20-35 g in body with 70% combined with calcium and phosphorus in bone; the remainder found in body fluids and within the cells and muscles; eliminated in urine and feces
Overdose symptoms	More than 15 g/day: flushed feeling, muscular weakness, hypotension, diminished reflexes, perspiration, decreased urinary output, lethargy, hypermagnesemia
Deficiency symptoms	Hypomagnesemia, twitching, tremors, spacicity, restlessness, confusion

Persons at risk	Chronic alcoholism, cirrhosis of liver, malabsorption, malnutrition, dehydration, diuretics, renal failure, antacids and laxatives containing magnesium, diabetes mellitus
Antagonists	Excess fat, phosphates, oxalic and phylic acids
Synergists	Acidic environment, potassium
Comments	Absorption in the small intestine
	High intake of calcium increases requirement of magnesium
	Diuretics can decrease reabsorption by the kidneys and digoxin can increase excretion of magnesium
	Use of antacids containing magnesium can cause chronic diarrhea

Iron (Fe)

RDA	10 mg/day for males and females
Principle sources	Fish, shellfish, beef, lamb, pork, veal, liver, kidney, ham, poultry, legumes, spinach, broccoli, green beans, cabbage, dried fruits, nuts, oats, barley, wheat germ, noodles
Function in body	Uptake and release of oxygen at cellular level and energy production
Storage in body	4 g iron in the body with the majority found in the hemoglobin of erythrocytes and 1 g stored in liver and spleen; the remainder stored in cells ready for use; losses occur in sweat, hair, urine and sloughing of epithelial and mucosa; bleeding and trauma add to iron loss

Overdose symptoms	More than 100 mg/day: poor liver function, diabetes from pancreas dysfunction, bronze skin, arrhythmias
Deficiency symptoms	Anemia with weakness, fatigue, pallor, dyspnea, tachycardia
Persons at risk	Malabsorption disorders, chronic blood loss, chronic renal failure, cancer of gastrointestinal tract, high altitudes
Antagonists	Tea, phosphates, oxalates and phytates, increased fluid intake
Synergists	Absorbic acid, fructose, sulfhydryl compounds, copper, acidic environment
Comments	Absorption in the small intestine; is influenced by type of foods ingested, body stores and needs, and gastric acidity
	Present in foods in form of heme or nonheme iron with heme iron found in animal tissues and nonheme in vegetable sources

Iodine (I)

RDA	150 µg/day for males and females
Principle sources	Seafoods, eggs, iodized salt
Function in body	Synthesis of iodinated thyroid hormones to regulate oxidation within the cells affecting temperature, metabolism, nerve and muscle tissue
Storage in body	20-50 mg in body with 1/3 stored in the thyroid gland and the remainder in skin, muscles, skeleton, and endocrine tissue

Overdose symptoms	More than 2,000 µg/day: hyperthyroidism, goiter, hyperactivity, hypermetabolism
Deficiency symptoms	Hypothyroidism: myxedema, hypofunction, mental and physical sluggishness
Persons at risk	Thyroiditis, protein malnutrition, pituitary dysfunction, hepatitis
Antagonists	Brussel sprouts, cabbage, cauliflower, peanuts are considered goitergens but effect is inactivated by cooking
Synergists	Thyroid stimulating hormone (TSH)
Comments	Absorbed as inorganic iodide after digestive process and transported in blood as free iodide or protein bound (PBD); TSH causes uptake of iodide by thyroid gland where it becomes part of thyroglobulin complex

Zinc (Zn)

RDA	15 mg/day for males and 12 mg/day for females
Principle sources	Meats, poultry, eggs, seafoods, vegetables
Function in body	Wound healing and tissue repair
	Enzyme activity for utilization of vitamin A, transfer of carbon dioxide, production of peptides and protein metabolism, conversion of pyruvic acid to lactic acid, and action of insulin
	Gustatory acuity

Storage in body	1.4-2.3 g in the body with 20% in the skin and the remainder in bones, teeth, liver, pancreas, brain, prostate, and kidneys
Overdose symptoms	More than 2 g/day: gastrointestinal irritation and vomiting
Deficiency symptoms	Anorexia, skin changes, impaired wound healing, decreased taste and smell
Persons at risk	Alcoholism, malabsorption syndromes, chronic renal failure, hyperalimentation, living in area where soil is deficient in zinc
Antagonists	High intake of fiber, calcium, and phytate
Synergists	Vitamin A
Comments	40% absorbed in the small intestine

Copper (Cu)

RDA	Recommended intake/day 1.5-3.0 mg/day for males and females
Principle sources	Oysters, nuts, shellfish, liver, kidneys, legumes, raisins
Function in body	Bone development
	Formation of hemoglobin, melanin pigment
	Synthesis of phospholipids
	Maintain nervous system myelin
	Energy production
	Purine metabolism and fatty acid oxidation
	Iron metabolism

Storage in body	100-150 mg in body at all times with a higher concentration in the liver and brain; eliminated in the feces
Overdose symptoms	More than 250 mg/day: anemia, thyroid dysfunction, hypercuperemia
Deficiency symptoms	Hypocuperemia, hypothennia, depigmentation of hair and skin, cerebral degeneration
	Wilson's disease, bone disease, protein malnutrition
Persons at risk	Use of penicillamine, long-term total parenteral nutrition, sprue, malabsorption syndromes, renal diseases, cirrhosis of liver, thyroid dysfunction, leukemias, anemia
Antagonists	Penicillamine
Synergists	Iron, zinc, molybdenum
Comments	Absorbed by stomach and small intestine
	Majority is bound to protein and small amount to albumin and amino acids
	Does not exist in free form

Manganese (Mn)

RDA	Recommended intake/day 2.0-5.0 mg/day for males and females
Principle sources	Tea, legumes, whole grains, nuts, fruits, vegetables
Function in body	Protein and energy metabolism
	Synthesis of cartilage, prothrombin, and gluconeogenesis

Storage in body	12-20 mg in the body mostly in liver and kidneys; excreted in feces with bile
Overdose symptoms	More than 1 g/day: neuromuscular disturbances
Deficiency symptoms	Abnormal formation of bone and cartilage, possible impaired glucose tolerance
Persons at risk	Poor dietary intake, malnutrition
Antagonists	None known
Synergists	Magnesium
Comments	Absorbed from the small intestine but main sites of uptake are the mitochondria

Selenium (Se)

RDA	70 µg/day for males and 55 µg/day for females
Principle sources	Seafoods, liver, kidneys, whole grains
Function in body	Immune activity
	Synthesis of ATP
	Antioxidant, cell protection
Storage in body	Highest concentrations in liver, pancreas, kidneys, and pituitary gland; excreted in the feces
Overdose symptoms	More than 0.4 µg/day can produce symptoms in animals
Deficiency symptoms	None in humans
Persons at risk	Related to dietary intake of meats and water containing Se
Antagonists	Sulfur
Synergists	None known

Comments	Absorbed in the intestine
	Content in food depends on concentration in soil

Electrolytes

Any substance that can dissociate into its component ions in a fluid is an electrolyte. Cations carry a positive charge (+) and anions carry a negative charge (-). In the body fluids, these are equal. Their unit of measurement is the milliequivalent (mEq). Cations are sodium, calcium, magnesium, and potassium. Anions are chloride, phosphate, sulfate, bicarbonate, and organic acids. Dietary intake is the source of electrolytes in the body. The major electrolytes (sodium, chloride, potassium) are covered in this section.

Sodium (Na)

RDA	Minimum recommended intake 500 mg/day for males and females
Principle sources	Table salt (NaCl), processed foods, cheese, crackers, processed meats, foods with additives or preservatives
Function in body	Principal cation, found in extracellular fluid
	Regulate acid-base balance in combination with chloride and bicarbonate
	Maintain osmotic pressure of fluids
	Maintain muscle activity and cell permeability
Storage in body	63 g in body, 1/3 of total in bones, and the remainder in extracellular fluid; excreted in urine and sweat

Overdose symptoms	More than 18 g/day or 30 g/day as NaCl: (hypernatremia), hypertension, edema
Deficiency symptoms	Fluid losses, dehydration (hyponatremia)
Persons at risk	Renal diseases, hypertension, vomiting, diarrhea, Addison's disease, taking several prescription medications
Antagonists	None
Synergists	Chloride, bicarbonate
Comments	1 tsp salt or 5 g = 2,000 mg Na
	Na intake should be limited to 2,400 mg/day
	Absorbed in the ileum
	Decreased Na intake causes increased aldosterone secretion and vice versa
	Decreased ability to adapt to Na intake and Na conservation in the older adult as there is a decrease in circulating renin and aldosterone

Chloride (Cl-)

RDA	Recommended intake/day 750 mg/day for males and females
Principle sources	Table salt (NaCl)
Function in body	Regulate osmotic pressure, fluid balance, acid-base balance
	Produce hydrochloric acid
	Assist blood to carry carbon dioxide to lungs

	Conserve potassium
	Anion found in extracellular fluid
Storage in body	85 g in body with 15% chloride mostly concentrated in cerebro-spinal fluid and gastrointestinal secretions, least amounts in muscle and nerve tissue with excretion in the urine
Overdose symptoms	Same as sodium and occur at the same time as for sodium
Deficiency symptoms	Fluid losses, dehydration
Persons at risk	Endocrine disorders, diarrhea, loss of gastric secretions during decompression, vomiting, profuse sweating
Antagonists	None
Synergists	Sodium, potassium
Comments	Absorbed in intestine

Potassium (K)

RDA	Recommended intake/day 3,500 mg/day for males and females
Principle sources	Chicken, veal, beef, pork, liver, dried fruits, citrus fruits, green and yellow vegetables
Function in body	Principal cation found in intracellular fluid
	Influence muscle activity including heart muscle
	Control blood pressure
	Synthesis of protein

	Maintain acid-base balance and osmotic pressure
	Contribute to enzyme activity
Storage in body	150 g in body with 30 times more concentration in the intracellular than in extracellular fluid with excretion in the urine
Overdose symptoms	More than 12 g/day: bradycardia, oliguria, (hyperkalemia), paresthesia, tingling and twitching of extremities, abdominal cramps, apprehension
Deficiency symptoms	Hypotension, vertigo, nausea, vomiting, (hypokalemia), diarrhea, muscle weakness, leg cramping, arrhythmias, confusion, depression, irritability
Persons at risk	Diuretic therapy, diarrhea, laxative, diabetic acidosis, malnutrition
Antagonists	None
Synergists	None
Comments	Absorbed in the intestine
	Kidneys are the major regulatory mechanism for potassium balance and changes related to aging can affect this balance
	Diuretic use is the most common cause of hypokalemia; impaired renal function or the administration of potassium replacement is the most likely cause of hyperkalemia in the older adult

Calculation of Caloric Content/Needs

The daily caloric requirements recommended for the older adult by the Food and Nutrition Board of the National Research Council are as follows:

Women (WT of 65 kg)	Men (WT of 77 kg)

Age 51-75

Total Energy Allowance (Based on moderate activity):

1,900 kcal/day	2,300 kcal/day

Resting Energy Expenditure (REE):

1,280 kcal/day	1,530 kcal/day

Range Allowable for Individual Variations:

1,520-2,280 kcal/day (plus or minus 20%)	1,840-2,760 kcal/day (plus or minus 20%)

Age 76 and over

1,600 calories/day or a reduction of 20% of the mature adult.	2,050 calories/day or a reduction of 20% of the mature adult.

Resting energy expenditure (REE) can be estimated for use in meal planning. Calculation is based on age and weight using the following formula:

Men > 60 years of age

REE in kcal/day = (13.5 x wt in kg) + 487

Women > 60 years of age

REE in kcal/day = (10.5 x wt in kg) + 596

Energy requirements for the older adult are based on caloric intake needed for optimal health and functional level. Maintenance levels should be considered separately.

The established energy value for the fuel producing nutrients are:

> Protein 4 kcal/g
>
> Carbohydrate 4 kcal/g
>
> Fat 9 kcal/g

If the composition of the food is known, the kcal is calculated as follows:

> 1 cup whole milk composed of 9 g protein, 12 g carbohydrate, 9 g fat
>
> 9 x4 = 36
>
> 12 x 4 – 48
>
> 9 x 9 = 81

Total   165 kcal (in 1 cup of whole milk)

A chart of foods and their contents is used to find the composition amounts of each nutrient in a measured amount of food. This is then calculated for kcal.

In most instances, however, these calculations are not necessary, as books with food values are used to determine caloric composition.

To calculate the amount of calories needed, the height, weight, and age are used to determine the basal energy expenditure (BEE) that is measured in calories/day.

Height is converted into centimeters (cm) using the equivalency:

> 1 inch (in) = 2.54 cm
>
> therefore, a 5 ft person = 5 ft x 12 in = 60 in
>
> and then, 60 in x 2.54 cm = 152.4 cm for a 5 ft person

Weight is converted into kilograms (kg) using the equivalency:

> 1 kg = 2.2 pounds (lb)
>
> therefore, a 105 lb person (105 lb ÷ 2.2 kg = 48.1)= 48.1 kg

The formula to calculate BEE for the male:

> 66 + (13.7 x wt in kg) + (5 x ht in cm)- (6.8 x age)

The formula to calculate BEE for the female:

$$655 + (9.6 \times \text{wt in kg}) + (1.8 \times \text{ht in cm}) - (4.7 \times \text{age})$$

Using the formula above, the calculation for caloric needs for a women 70 years of age who is 5 ft tall (152.4 cm) and weighs 105 lb (48.1 kg) is:

$$655 + (9.6 \times 48.1 \text{ kg}) + (1.8 \times 152.4 \text{ cm}) - (4.7 \times 70)$$

$$655 + (461.76) + (274.32) - (329)$$

BEE = 1,062.08 or 1,062 calories/day required
for body at rest

The formula to estimate BEE:

1 cal/kg/hour for males

0.9 cal/kg/hour for females

Using the estimate formula for the same person:

0.9 cal $\times$ 48.1 kg = 43.29 cal/hour

43.29 cal $\times$ 24 hours = 1,038.96 or 1,039 cal/day

An estimate of the desired weight of a person with a medium frame that is underweight or overweight is calculated using a formula as follows:

	Male	Female
First 5 ft of height	106 lb	100 lb
Added for every additional inch	6 lb	5 lb

10% of total body weight is added for a person with a large frame

10% of total body weight is subtracted for a person with a small frame

Using the above formula for a large framed male who is 5 ft 9 in and weighs 170 lb, the desired weight is calculated as follows:

Desired wt = 106 + (9 $\times$ 6)

106 + 54

Desired wt = 160 lb for medium frame

The adjustment for a large male is as follows:

> 10% of 160 lb (.1 x 160)= 16 lb
>
> Desired wt = 160 + 16
>
> Desired wt = 176 lb
>
> This person is 6 lb overweight

Suggested Weights For Adults

This table may be used instead of the above calculations:

Height[1]	Weight in Pounds[2]	
	19 to 34 years	35 years and over
5'0"	97-128	108-138
5'1"	101-132	111-143
5'2"	104-137	115-148
5'3"	107-141	119-152
5'4"	111-146	122-157
5'5"	114-150	126-162
5'6"	118-155	130-167
5'7"	121-160	134-172
5'8"	125-164	138-178
5'9"	129-169	142-183
5'10"	132-174	146-188
5'11"	136-179	151-194
6'0"	140-184	155-199
6'1"	144-189	159-205
6'2"	148-195	164-210
6'3"	152-200	168-216
6'4"	156-205	173-222
6'5"	160-211	177-228
6'6"	164-216	182-234

[1] Without shoes

[2] Without clothes

[3] The higher weights in the ranges generally apply to men, who tend to have more muscle and bone; the lower weights more often apply to women, who have less muscle and bone.

Source: U.S. Department of Health and Human Services. National Institutes of Health. NIH Publication No. 94-3680. November 1993.

Calculation of Fluid Needs

Total body water content decreases with age. In young males, 60% of total body weight is water compared to 50% in the older adult male. In young females, 52% of total weight is water compared to 46% in the older adult female. The normal adult gains and loses approximately 2,400 mL fluids/day and the ratio between the intake and output (I&O) determines the risk for or actual presence of fluid disturbances. Body fluids are obtained from ingestion of liquids, liquids in foods, and oxidation of proteins, carbohydrates, and fats. Fluids are mainly eliminated by excretion from the kidneys that also have the ability to conserve water when needed to prevent imbalances. Serious fluid and electrolyte imbalances can occur rapidly in the older adult from tube feedings, intravenous therapy, malnutrition, and with the use of diuretics or laxatives. Also, impairments associated with the older adult can affect fluid balance, e.g., reduced thirst mechanism, reduced ability to conserve water by the kidneys, decreased intake caused by inability to obtain fluids without assistance. The average amounts and routes of fluid losses and gains are as follows:

Fluid Losses/Day		Fluid Gains/Day	
800-1,500 mL	Urine	1,000-1,250 mL	Oral liquids
250-350 mL	Feces	600-1,250 mL	Foods
100-250 mL	Perspiration	200-400 mL	Metabolic oxidation
250-350 mL	Skin (Insensible)		
350 mL	Lungs		
1,900-2,800 mL	*Total Losses/Day*	1,850-2,900 mL	*Total Gains/Day*
Other losses	Tears, vomiting, diarrhea, wound, exudate, suction, hemorrhage	**Other gains**	Tube feeding, parenteral feeding and/or fluid

Weight is usually used in the calculation of fluid needs for 24 hours.

Calculation for the amount of fluid needed by a person is as follows:

> Allow 100 mL/kg for the first 10 kg (22 lb) of body weight
>
> Add 50 mL/kg for the next 10 kg body weight
>
> After the first 20 kg (44 lb), add 15 mL/kg body weight

For a 78 kg (167 lb) person:

> 100 mL x 10 kg = 1,000 mL
>
> 50 mL x 10 kg = 500 mL
>
> 15 mL x 56 kg = 840 mL
>
> 1,000 mL + 500 mL + 840 mL = 2,340 mL/day Total

Another method to estimate fluid needs for 24 hours is as follows:

Allow 1,000 mL for every 1,000 kcal in 24 hour dietary intake

For a person receiving a 1,800 kcal diet:

> 1,000 mL= 1,000 kcal
>
> 800 mL = 800 kcal
>
> 1,000 mL + 800 mL = 1,800 mL/day Total

Fluids are generally replaced during the day and amounts can be scheduled for administration during the 3 shifts in 24 hours in a long-term facility as follows:

7AM-3PM shift	1/2 of total calculated 24 hour fluids
3PM-11PM shift	1/3 of total calculated 24 hour fluids
11PM-7AM shift	1/6 of total calculated 24 hour fluids

Scheduling can be modified for an individual as some older adults do better with fluid intake spread over daytime hours with ingestion of 100-150 mL/hour. Avoid fluid intake prior to bedtime or during the night.

To increase fluids, the 24 hour amount should be doubled, but for the older adult, increases should occur slowly over a period of time in order to avoid a fluid overload. This does not mean, however, that the older adult should not be treated for dehydration as vigorously as a person of any age.

Chapter V

DIETS AND MENUS

A. Clear Liquid
B. Blenderized Liquid
C. Low Residue/Bland
D. Mechanical Soft
E. Pureed Soft/Blenderized
F. General
G. High Fiber
H. Low Caloric/Reduction
I. High Caloric/High Protein
J. Iron Rich
K. Protein Restricted
L. Low Fat/Cholesterol
M. Low Sodium
N. High Potassium
O. Potassium Restricted

Clear Liquid Diet

Indications	Acute illness and infection
	Preoperative care
	Postoperative care
	Step #1 from NPO to Regular Diet
	Temporary food intolerance
	Preparation for a laboratory test or diagnostic procedure
Restrictions	Solid or pureed foods
	Milk and milk products
	Carbonated beverages
	Fruit juices with pulp
Inclusions	Ginger ale, fruit flavored drinks
	Water, tea, decaffeinated coffee
	Clear fruit juices, lemonade
	Popsicles, plain gelatin
	Broth, bouillon, consommé
	Hard clear candies, honey, sugar
Comments	Limited nutritional value
	Deficient in protein, minerals, calories, and vitamins
	Provides fluids and relieves thirst
Additional Interventions	Offer fluids frequently, q 1-2 hour intervals
	Avoid exposure to more advanced diets at mealtimes

Sample Clear Liquid Diet

Breakfast	Cereal beverage
	Apple or cranberry juice
	Coffee, tea, and sugar/honey
Mid-Morning	Ginger ale
Lunch	Clear broth
	Clear, flavored gelatin
	Strained fruit juice
	Tea, coffee, and sugar/honey

Mid-Afternoon	Popsicle
Dinner	Fruit flavored drink
	Consommé
	Plain, clear gelatin
	Tea, coffee, with sugar/honey
	Clear sugar candy
Evening	Grape juice

Blenderized Liquid Diet

Indications	Acute gastritis and infections
	Step #2 from NPO to Regular Diet
	Febrile conditions
	Chewing or swallowing dysfunction
	Extreme weakness
	Dehydration
Restrictions	Solid or pureed foods
Inclusions	All items included in
	Clear Liquid Diet
	Milk, milk drinks
	Noncarbonated beverages
	Strained fruit and vegetable juices
	Cooked refined cereals/gruel
	Custard, pudding, ice cream, sherbet
	Creamed soups
	Butter, margarine, cream
Comments	Inclusions are foods that are liquid at room temperature
	All foods may be blenderized to a liquid form as tolerated
Additional Interventions	Offer 6 feedings/day or 2-4 hour feeding intervals
	Offer fluids frequently
	Advance to Regular Diet as soon as possible for complete nutritional requirement intake

Sample Blenderized Liquid Diet

Breakfast	Strained orange juice Oatmeal thinned with milk Milk or eggnog Coffee, tea, with cream and sugar/honey
Mid-Morning	Sherbet or thin milkshake
Lunch	Tomato juice Cream of potato soup Pureed beef thinned with broth Pureed green beans thinned with chicken broth Vanilla ice cream Milk, coffee, tea, with cream/sugar
Mid-Afternoon	Flavored yogurt
Dinner	Cranberry juice Cream of chicken soup with pureed chicken Mashed potato thinned with milk Pudding Milk, coffee, tea, with cream/sugar
Evening	Hot cocoa or milk shake Blenderized fruit thinned with orange juice

Low Residue/Bland Diet

Indications	Indigestion, esophageal reflux Colitis, irritable bowel, gastritis, diverticular disease, diarrhea Chemotherapy/Radiation therapy
Restrictions	Milk and milk products limited Alcohol, fruit juices with pulp Raw fruits and vegetables and those with skin Coconut, raisins Nuts, seeds, condiments Rich or spicy gravies, sauces

All fried foods, hot breads
Jams, yogurt with fresh fruit
Coarse cereals and whole grain breads
Peanut butter
Smoked, pickled, or cured meats
Rich desserts (pies, cakes, cobblers)
Corn, onions, dried beans, peas

Inclusions

All beverages except alcohol
White bread, rolls, crackers
Rice, noodles, macaroni, spaghetti
Cooked cereals, dry cereal without bran
Cottage, cheddar, American cheese
Lean, tender, ground, broiled, baked, or stewed meats, chicken or turkey without skin, liver, all eggs but fried
Crisp bacon, canned tuna or salmon
Broth, cream and vegetable soup
Butter, margarine, cream, oil, mayonnaise
Tender cooked vegetables, vegetable juices
Strained fruit juices, ripe banana, applesauce, skinless stewed or canned fruits
Custards, puddings, sherbet, plain ice cream, angel food or sponge cake, plain cookies
Sugar, vinegar, lemon juice, spices as tolerated

Comments

Hot and cold foods should be eaten slowly
Milk products, if taken, limited to 2 cups/daily
Diet reduces amount of fecal material in the lower bowel

Additional Interventions	Food tolerances and preferences must have high priority in selections
	Offer 6 small meals/day to avoid distention
	Evening feeding can be eliminated to reduce acid secretion during the night

Sample Low Residue/Bland Diet

Breakfast	Cranapple juice
	Cooked oatmeal with cream/milk
	Scrambled egg
	Slice white toast with margarine
	Coffee, tea, with cream/sugar
Mid-Morning	Milk shake
Lunch	Chicken breast, baked
	White bread or roll
	Mashed potato
	Tender asparagus with margarine
	Ripe banana, sugar cookies
	Milk, tea, with cream/sugar
Mid-Afternoon	Plain yogurt
Dinner	Baked trout
	Rice, buttered
	Cooked carrots
	White bread with margarine/butter
	Custard
	Coffee, tea, with cream/sugar
Evening	Applesauce, or slice of angel food cake

Mechanical Soft Diet

Indications	Chewing, swallowing difficulties
	Poor dentition, poor fitting dentures
	Head and neck surgery; anatomical esophageal strictures

Restrictions	Fried foods
	Franks, sausages, pork chops, chili with beans
	Most raw fruits and vegetables, foods with nuts, seeds
	Citrus fruit, pineapple
	Pulpy fruits, prunes, fruits with skins, dried fruit
Inclusions	All beverages
	White, whole wheat, rye bread without seeds, saltine and graham crackers
	Cooked or prepared refined cereals
	Plain cakes, cookies, puddings, custards, smooth ice cream, sherbet, gelatin, fruit slushes
	Butter, margarine, vegetable oil salad dressings, white sauce
	All fruit juices, cooked or canned fruits without skins, ripe banana
	Egg, chopped, ground, pureed, or tender meats and poultry, casseroles
	Cream, cottage, mild cheddar cheese
	Broth and cream soups, soups with soft vegetables
	Potatoes, hominy, rice, spaghetti, noodles, macaroni
	All vegetable juices, cooked or canned tender vegetables
	Sugar, honey, syrup, clear jelly/jam
Comments	Offer any soft, chopped, ground, pureed foods with a moist consistency
	Nutritionally adequate diet
	Restrict food preparation and seasoning according to individual needs
	Avoid any inclusions that give rise to difficulty in chewing, swallowing, or use of facial muscles

Additional Interventions	Offer 6 feedings/day or 3 meals with between meal feedings
	Encourage to eat food in bite-sized amounts at one time
	Allow time, avoid rushing through meals
	Foods with texture are easier to control in the mouth and swallow
	Position upright for meals

Sample Mechanical Soft Diet

Breakfast	Orange juice
	Farina with milk
	Soft cooked egg
	Whole wheat toast with margarine/jelly
	Milk, coffee, tea, with cream/sugar

| Mid-Morning | Fruit slush |

Lunch	Vegetable soup/saltines
	Tender roast beef
	Baked potato
	Buttered spinach
	Tomato juice
	Slice white bread with margarine
	Smooth ice cream
	Milk or milk shake

| Mid-Afternoon | Eggnog or yogurt |

Dinner	Baked white fish, plain or with cream sauce
	Tender cooked seasoned carrots
	Slice whole wheat bread with margarine
	Canned pears
	Slice sponge cake
	Milk, coffee, tea, with cream/sugar

| Evening | Plain cookies or pudding |

Pureed Soft/Blenderized Diet

The following are general guidelines and are not sufficient to the nutrition management of dysphagia. Neurologic illnesses, surgical or radiation treatments, as well as aging may lead to dysphagia and risk for aspiration. If dysphagia is suspected, a swallowing evaluation by a qualified speech-language pathologist should be completed. An individualized dietary prescription is then developed in conjunction with the dietitian which will specify appropriate level of thinness and texture for all foods and fluids.

Indications

Chewing, swallowing difficulties
Tooth loss or tooth/gum pain
Poor fitting dentures
Stomatitis
Gastrointestinal disorders/diseases
Extreme weakness

Restrictions

All fried, spicy, and gas-forming foods

Inclusions

Milk, milk drinks, egg if not fried
Carbonated beverages, fruit drinks
Coffee, tea, decaffeinated coffee
White toast, saltine and graham cracker
Cooked or prepared refined cereals
Custard, pudding, ice cream, sherbet, gelatin, popsicles
Plain cake and cookies
Fruit slushes, fruit juices, ripe banana, vegetable juices
Pureed cooked or canned fruit and vegetables
Butter, margarine, cream, vegetable oils, salad dressings, white sauce
Broths and cream soups with pureed vegetables and meats
Pureed or finely ground beef, lamb, veal, chicken, turkey, lean pork, fish in broth or cream sauce
Cream, cottage, and other mild cheese

	Mashed potato, rice, noodles, hominy, spaghetti Honey, sugar, syrup, jelly, clear hard candy
Comments	Food consistency dependent on appetite, ability to chew, dysphagia
Additional Interventions	Offer 6 feedings/day Encourage to take small amounts of food at one time Allow time, avoid rushing through meal Place in upright position Encourage to participate in communal meals

Sample Pureed Soft/Blenderized Diet

Breakfast	Orange juice Corn flakes or puffed rice with milk Soft cooked egg Slice white toast with margarine/jelly Milk, coffee, tea, with cream/sugar
Mid-Morning	Chocolate milk shake
Lunch	Strained vegetable soup Ground chicken pattie Mashed white potato Pureed carrots, V-8 juice Slice white bread with margarine/butter Custard Milk, coffee, tea, with cream/sugar
Mid-Afternoon	Ice cream or fruit slush
Dinner	Creamed, ground beef sirloin on noodles Pureed green beans Slice white bread with margarine/butter

Pureed peaches with slice angel
food cake
Milk, coffee, tea, with cream/sugar

Evening   Eggnog or 2 graham crackers

General Diet

Indications   Ambulatory individuals
                                   Ability to eat and tolerate any food
                                   or food combinations

Restrictions   Fried foods in moderation
                                   Spices and pastries in moderation
                                   Modifications in prescribed
                                   therapeutic diets

Inclusions   All foods permitted

Comments   Normal, adequate,
                                   well-balanced diet

Additional Interventions   Allow as much time as needed
                                   for meals
                                   Provide assistive aids for self-
                                   feeding if appropriate
                                   Assist with eating or feed as needed
                                   Provide sufficient fluid

Sample General Diet

Breakfast   Grapefruit
                                   Oatmeal with milk
                                   Banana, whole wheat toast with
                                   margarine, jelly
                                   Milk, coffee, tea, with cream/sugar

Lunch   Beef, vegetable soup
                                   Turkey/tomato/lettuce, club
                                   sandwich on toast with
                                   salad dressing
                                   Creamed potatoes
                                   Buttered peas
                                   Gelatin
                                   Milk

Mid-Afternoon	Graham crackers/milk
Dinner	Broiled chicken breast
	Sweet potato
	Lettuce salad with dressing
	Cauliflower
	Whole wheat bread with
	margarine/butter
	Slice angel food cake with fruit
	Milk, coffee, tea, with cream/sugar
Evening	Fruit or fruit yogurt

High Fiber Diet

Indications	Constipation, diverticular disease
	Possibly to lower cholesterol levels
Restrictions	Refined foods and grains
Inclusions	6 or more servings of the following:
	Whole wheat/grain breads, crackers
	Bran type cereals, oatmeal, shredded
	wheat, wheat germ
	Wild rice, cornmeal, buckwheat,
	groats, barley
	2 or more servings:
	Fresh fruits with skins, dried fruit
	3 or more servings:
	Raw and slightly steamed
	vegetables
	Legumes, nuts, seeds, popcorn
	Oatmeal, bran, raisin
	muffins/cookies
Comments	High fiber intake will stimulate
	peristalsis and promote bowel
	evacuation without straining
	Dietary fiber refers to all
	undigestible carbohydrates
	and lignin from plants

Additional Interventions	Increase daily fluid intake to 8-10 glasses/day and encourage activity Fiber is usually added to General Diet Recommended daily intake of fiber is 25-30 g and is derived from plant sources

Sample High Fiber Diet

Breakfast	Grapefruit sections Raisin all-bran cereal with milk Whole wheat toast (2) Margarine, jam Milk, coffee, tea, with cream/sugar
Mid-Morning	Apple
Lunch	Split pea soup Sliced chicken/lettuce/tomato sandwich on whole wheat bread with mayonnaise Chef salad Oatmeal cookies Milk, coffee, tea, with cream/sugar
Mid-Afternoon	Banana nut bread slice or dried fruit
Dinner	Roast beef Baked potato with skin Fresh fruit salad Green beans Bran muffin with margarine/butter Strawberries Milk, coffee, tea, with cream/sugar
Evening	Raisin cookies or fresh pear

Low Caloric/Reduction Diet (1,200 Calorie)

Indications	More than 20% over normal weight for height, weight and frame, BMI >25 Maintenance of desired weight
Restrictions	All fried foods Butter, margarine, oils, creams, gravies limited Desserts and sweets such as candy, ice cream, cakes, pies, sugar in beverages or foods
Inclusions	All foods allowed on a General Diet with exchanges for low caloric foods in each food group Low fat dairy products, fat trimmed meats, sugar free foods and beverages Raw and cooked fruits and vegetables
Comments	Food servings should be reduced Artificial sweeteners and spices can be used for flavoring Caloric content can be from 1,000-1,600 calories/day
Additional Interventions	Include a regular exercise program for successful weight loss Eat regular meals, avoid skipping meals Measure portion of food Bake, broil, or steam foods

Sample Low Caloric/Reduction Diet

Breakfast	1/4 cantaloupe 1 scrambled egg 1 slice whole wheat toast 1 tsp margarine 1/2 cup farina 1 cup low fat/skim milk Coffee, tea

Lunch	1/2 cup tuna (water packed)
	2 slices white bread
	Lettuce, cucumber, tomato salad
	with vinegar or lemon juice
	1/2 banana
	Coffee, tea, or diet soda
Dinner	3 oz baked chicken without skin
	1 medium baked potato with
	1 tsp margarine
	1/2 cup cooked carrots
	Green tossed salad
	2 fresh plums
	1 cup low fat/skim milk
Snack	Fresh apple
	Dietetic gelatin

High Caloric/High Protein Diet

Indications	Hypermetabolic states
	Chronic wasting illnesses
	(cancer, COPD)
	Malnutrition
Restrictions	No foods restricted
	Avoid foods that increase nausea
	and vomiting such as greasy, strong
	odorous, rich or sweet foods
	Avoid drinking fluids with meals
Inclusions	All foods allowed on General Diet
	with exchanges for high caloric and
	protein foods in each group
	Addition of margarine, powdered
	milk to sauces, gravies, soups, hot
	cereals
	Eggs, casseroles, rice, potatoes,
	pancakes, breads
	Use milk instead of water in
	preparing foods
	Add meats to noodles, soups, and
	rice casseroles
	Add cheese to noodles, vegetables,
	soups, rice, and sauces

	Add mayonnaise or salad dressing to eggs, sandwiches, and salads Spread peanut butter on bread, cookies, vegetables, fruits Add nuts to breads, cookies, cakes, ice cream or as a snack Add honey to toast, cereals, coffee, tea Add whipped cream on desserts; sour cream or yogurt to vegetables Dressings, potatoes, gravies
Comments	Increase amounts in food servings Anorexia, altered taste and smell sensations affect food intake All high caloric and protein foods can be exchanged for usual foods eaten
Additional Interventions	Encourage to eat regular meals, avoid skipping meals Offer frequent meals, 4-6/day Encourage between meal snacks Provide commercially prepared supplemental drinks with medications Monitor weight and praise accomplishments in weight gains Do not offer supplements during meals

Sample High Caloric/High Protein Diet

Breakfast	Large orange juice 2 poached or scrambled eggs 2 slices toast with margarine/jelly Oatmeal made with fortified milk 1 cup high protein milk Coffee, tea, with cream/sugar
Mid-Morning	Custard or yogurt

Lunch	Cheeseburger with lettuce/tomato
	Mashed potatoes made with
	fortified milk
	Fresh peach and grapes with honey
	1 cup milk
Mid-Afternoon	Fruit and cottage cheese
Dinner	Creamed vegetable soup
	Pork chop with applesauce
	Seasoned noodles
	Asparagus salad with mayonnaise
	Roll and margarine
	Tapioca pudding with whipped
	topping
	1 glass high protein enriched milk
Evening	Crackers and peanut butter
	Juice

Iron Rich Diet

Indications	Iron deficiency anemia
	Diseases that interfere with iron
	absorption
Restrictions	No foods are restricted
Inclusions	Emphasis on animal proteins,
	enriched breads and cereals
Comments	Iron is needed for synthesis
	of hemoglobin
	Most iron is supplied by the meat
	group followed by the bread and
	cereal groups
Additional Interventions	Foods can be selected from
	General Diet menus
	Iron rich foods should be taken in
	combination with vitamin C foods

Sample Iron Rich Diet

Breakfast	Orange juice Oatmeal Enriched white toast with margarine Poached egg or omelet Milk, coffee, tea, with cream/sugar
Mid-Morning	Whole orange
Lunch	Sliced roast beef on 2 slices of enriched bread Cole slaw Canned pineapple
Mid-Afternoon	1 cup milk
Dinner	Roast pork Baked potato with margarine Spinach salad with dressing Seasoned peas Whole wheat bread Strawberry cake Coffee, tea, with cream/sugar
Evening	Stewed prunes/orange

Protein Restricted Diet (50 grams)

Indications	Renal disease, hepatic failure
Restrictions	Protein foods, mainly meats, eggs, and milk products Fats and Na, K, P can also be restricted with low protein diets
Inclusions	Foods low in protein with protein derived from high biological value sources Foods high in caloric value
	Hard candies, coffee, tea Apples, berries, cherries, grapefruit, peaches, pears, pineapple, prunes Margarine, sour cream, oil

Comments	Specify daily protein amount in g and if other restrictions should be enforced
	Provide sufficient calories and nutrients daily
	Protein increases can be in 10 g/day increments as tolerated
	Multi-vitamins are often prescribed as diet may be low in B vitamins, calcium
	Protein is essential to health and cannot be eliminated for long periods of time
	Compliance is often difficult but necessary to reduce workload to kidneys or liver
Additional Interventions	Consider the possible need for other dietary restrictions
	Milk and eggs are primary sources of essential amino acids for diet inclusion of protein

Sample Protein Restricted Diet

Breakfast	Orange juice, 1/2 cup
	Corn flakes
	Whole wheat toast (2)
	*2 tsp margarine, jelly
	1/4 cup milk
	Coffee, tea, with cream/sugar
Mid-Morning	1/2 banana
Lunch	*1/4 cup tuna
	2 slices bread
	*2 tbsp mayonnaise
	Green salad with lemon/vinegar
	Gelatin with whipped topping
	Carbonated drink
	Baked apple
Mid-Afternoon	Hard candy or jelly beans

Dinner	2 oz baked chicken
	1/2 cup mashed potatoes
	*Peas with 1 tsp butter
	Fruit cocktail
	1/2 cup fruit drink
	Coffee, tea, with cream/sugar
Evening	Frozen pop

Salt-free foods can be used where applicable for renal or liver failure

Low Fat/Cholesterol Diet

Indications	Gallbladder, liver, or pancreatic diseases
	Cardiovascular disease
	High risk for atherosclerosis
	Overweight
Restrictions	All fried and fatty foods
	Biscuits, doughnuts, waffles, pancakes, french toast
	Avocados, olives, nuts
	Cheeses, whole milk, ice cream, cream
	Organ meats, skin of poultry, fatty meats, shrimp, luncheon meats
	Sauces, gravies, creams
	Butter, lard, high saturated oils
	Cakes, pastries containing egg
	No more than 3 eggs/week
Inclusions	Lean meats, poultry, fish that is baked, broiled, or steamed
	Cholesterol-free oils, margarine, dressings within fat restriction
Inclusions	All fruits and vegetables prepared and served without butter or toppings
	Skim milk, low fat/cholesterol cheese and yogurt, egg whites

	All breads, cakes made with minimal eggs and whole milk Legumes and pasta products without eggs
Comments	Low fat diet reduces gallbladder contractions and pain Fat is not added in preparing foods Seasonings improve the taste of foods Fat content is modified to increase ratio of polyunsaturated fatty acids to saturated fatty acids Calories can be modified if combined with a reduction diet
Additional Interventions	Diet can be low fat or low cholesterol and low saturated fat depending on underlying factors Many cholesterol-free products are available for food selections

Sample Low Fat/Cholesterol Diet

Breakfast	Orange juice Farina Low cholesterol scrambled egg Slice toast with margarine/jelly Skim milk Coffee, tea, with sugar/sweetener
Lunch	Skinless baked chicken Mashed potato with margarine Green salad with tomato and low fat/cholesterol dressing Slice bread Slice angel food cake Iced tea, coffee with sugar

Dinner	Lean hamburger pattie
	Hamburger bun
	Green beans with seasoning
	Rice with margarine/tomato sauce
	Peach and low cholesterol cottage cheese salad
	Watermelon
	Skim milk
Snacks	Whole apple
	Pudding made with skim milk

Low Sodium Diet

Indications	Renal diseases, fluid retention Hypertension, heart failure
Restrictions	Commercially prepared foods made with milk or milk products
	Canned vegetables or frozen products processed with sodium
	Potato chips, snack foods
	Vegetable or tomato juice
	Breads or commercial mixes made with salt, MSG, baking soda or powder
	Breads, rolls, crackers with salted tops
	Instant hot cereal
	Canned, smoked, salted meats, or fish
	Cold cuts, bacon
	Anchovies, herring, shellfish, sardines
	Commercial salad dressings unless low salt
	Pudding, cake, cookie and other types of mixes
	Pickles, olives, relish, soy sauce, sauerkraut, salted nuts

Inclusions	Skim and whole fresh milk Fresh, frozen, or canned fruits and vegetables without salt Enriched breads and cereals Meat, poultry, fish, eggs, low sodium cheese, and peanut butter Butter, margarine, cooking oils, and fats, low sodium salad dressing Jams, jellies, and syrup
Comments	1 mEq Na = 23 mg Totally salt free diet is impossible as sodium is found in most foods Restrictions should be specific as mild (2,500-4,500 mg/day), moderate (1,000-2,000 mg/day) Restriction below 2,000 mg is difficult and often impractical for long-term use
Additional Interventions	Salt or seasonings containing sodium are not added when preparing foods Remove salt shaker from the table or tray; avoid adding salt to prepared food Modify sodium allowance by restricting milk products (limit to 2 cups/day) and meats, using salt free foods as needed Use salt substitutes when possible Instruct to read all labels for sodium content

Sample Low Sodium Diet

Breakfast	1/2 cup orange juice 1/2 banana 3/4 cup whole grain cereal 1 cup milk *Slice toast and margarine/jelly Poached egg Coffee, tea, with sugar

Lunch	*Low sodium vegetable soup with unsalted crackers
	*Chicken salad sandwich with mayonnaise
	Green salad
	Fresh apple
	1/2 cup sherbet
	Iced tea, coffee
Dinner	Moderate portion of roast beef (3 oz)
	Medium sized baked potato
	Margarine or 1 tbsp sour cream
	1/2 cup beets
	1 roll
	*1 cup pudding or sherbet
	Coffee, tea, with sugar

*Use salt free foods

High Potassium Diet

Indications	Potassium loss with diuretic use
Restrictions	No restrictions
Inclusions	All fruits, especially citrus fruits Bananas, dates, raisins, prunes, melons All vegetables, especially broccoli, potatoes, legumes, brussel sprouts, parsnips, rhubarb Whole grain breads, bran cereals, wheat germ Meat, broth, bouillon Chocolate, molasses, nuts
Comments	Potassium replacement is necessary if blood level is too low High potassium foods may also contain sodium and must be regulated if on low sodium diet Hypokalemia results from fluid losses

Additional Interventions	Inform of signs and symptoms of hypokalemia such as malaise, anorexia, weak pulse, vomiting, decreased blood pressure and reflexes
	Increase in dietary intake of potassium depends on type of diuretic administered (potassium sparing)
	Many salt substitutes are made with potassium chloride and may be used

Sample High Potassium Diet

Breakfast	Large orange juice Fried egg Toast with butter/margarine/jelly Bran cereal Milk, coffee, tea, with cream/sugar
Lunch	Tuna salad sandwich on whole wheat bread Lettuce salad with dressing Banana Milk
Dinner	Meat loaf and gravy Baked potato with sour cream Broccoli Mixed salad with tomato and dressing Bran muffin Fresh fruit compote Coffee, tea, with cream/sugar
Evening	Hot cocoa made with milk Honeydew or watermelon

Potassium Restricted Diet

Indications	Renal diseases
Restrictions	Banana, cantaloupe, watermelon, grapefruit or orange juice, nectarine, potatoes, tomato and tomato juice, figs, avocado Artichokes, broccoli, collard, rutabaga, squash, legumes, soybeans Bran cereals Peanuts, raisins, prunes, dates
Inclusions	Lettuce, radishes, tomatoes, green pepper, green beans, asparagus, carrots Cranberry juice, lemons, canned peaches, blueberries, canned pears, fruit cocktail Breads, spaghetti, cornstarch, wheat starch, tapioca, rice, noodles Cottage cheese, eggs, chicken, meats, fish Canned foods that are drained Butter, fats, oils
Comments	5 mEq K = 200 mg Restrictions range from 1300-3,000 mg/day with a normal range of intake about 2,000-6,000 mg/day Amount of restriction should be specific in an ordered diet Diet is often combined with sodium and protein restricted diets Hyperkalemia is the result of kidney's inability to excrete potassium
Additional Interventions	Inform of signs and symptoms of hyperkalemia such as diarrhea, cramping, irritability, oliguria Inform to read labels for sodium content

Sample Potassium Restricted Diet

Breakfast	Cranberry juice cocktail Toast with margarine/jelly Poached egg Puffed rice Milk, coffee, tea, with sugar
Lunch	Sliced chicken sandwich on white bread Green salad with oil and vinegar Fruit cocktail Carbonated drink
Dinner	Meatballs and buttered noodles Green beans Cottage cheese and drained pineapple salad Lettuce salad with dressing Baked apple White dinner roll Coffee, tea, with sugar

CHAPTER VI

GENERAL FOOD EXCHANGE LISTS

A.   Food Group Exchanges
        Grain/Starch/Bread Exchanges
        Fruit Exchanges
        Milk Exchanges
        Vegetable Exchanges
        Meat Exchanges
        Fat Exchanges

B.   Cultural/Ethnic Exchanges
        Mexican American Selections
        African American Selections
        Asian Selections
        Italian Selections
        Mideastern Selections
        Jewish Selections
        Vegetarian Selections

FOOD GROUP EXCHANGES

Exchanges are used for meal planning to modify diets for those requiring special considerations or preferences because of disease or disabling disorders. The groups are divided according to the amount of protein, carbohydrate, fat, and calorie content in the food. The choices on the lists are approximately equal in order to allow for food exchanges when planning complete dietary menus. Approximate composition of a serving of each nutrient in grams (g) is:

Food	Protein	Carbohydrate	Fat	Calories
Starch/Bread	3	15	trace	80
Fruit	0	15	0	60
Milk				
Skim	8	12	trace	90
Low fat	8	12	5	120
Whole	8	12	8	150
Vegetable	2	5	0	25
Meat				
Lean	7	0	3	55
Medium fat	7	0	5	75
High fat	7	0	8	100
Fat	0	0	5	45

Grain/Starch/Bread Exchanges:

15 g carbohydrate, 3 g protein, 80 calories/exchange

Bread:

White, whole wheat, rye, pumpernickel	1 slice
Raisin bagel, English muffin, hamburger or hotdog bun	1/2
Plain roll	1
Bread crumbs	1 tbsp
Tortilla, pita	1

Cereal:

Cooked cereal, grits, rice, barley, pasta	1/2 cup
Dry bran flakes	1/2 cup
Puffed cereal (unfrosted)	1 1/2 cup
Ready-to-eat dry cereals	3/4 cup
Popcorn (plain)	3 cups
Wheat germ	3 tbsp
Flour	3 tbsp
Cornmeal	3 tbsp

Crackers:

Arrowroot	3
Graham, 2 1/2" square	3
Matzo	3/4
Oyster	24
Rye wafer	3
Saltines	6
Soda	4

Legumes:

Beans, peas, lentils (dried and cooked)	1/2 cup
Baked beans (canned, no pork)	1/3 cup

Starchy vegetables:

Corn	1/2 cup
Corn on cob	1 medium
Lima beans	2/3 cup
Winter squash	1 cup
Parsnips	2/3 cup
White potato	1 small
Pumpkin	3/4 cup
Sweet potato, yam	1/2 cup
Green peas, mashed potato	1/2 cup

Prepared Foods (count as 1 starch plus 1 fat):

Biscuit	1
Cornbread, cornbread muffin 2" cube	1
Muffin	1 small
Pancake, 4" across	2
Waffle	1
Potato or corn chips	15
French fried potatoes	8

Conditions using this modification:

Inclusion: Diabetes mellitus, malnutrition, all conditions with adjustments made for oral disorders, general diet, high caloric diet

Exclusion: Those foods with high fat, cholesterol, sodium content, clear and full liquid diets, reduced caloric/reduction diet, soft/low residue/bland diets except for toast and cooked cereals

Fruit Exchanges:

15 g carbohydrate, 60 calories/exchange

Apple, orange, pear, nectarine	1 small
Apple, pineapple juice, cider	1/2 cup
Applesauce (unsweetened)	1/2 cup
Apricots	4 whole
Banana, mango	1 small
Plums	2 medium
Prunes	3
Cherries	12
Grapes	17 small
Blackberries, blueberries, raspberries, pineapple	3/4 cup
Orange, grapefruit juice	1/2 cup
Prune, grape juice	1/3 cup
Dates	3
Peach	1 medium
Tangerines	2 small
Raisins	2 tbsp
Figs (fresh or dried)	2 medium
Strawberries	1 1/4 cup
Papaya	1 cup cubed
Watermelon	1 1/4 cup
Cantaloupe	1/3 small
Honeydew	1 cup cubed
Cranberries (unsweetened)	As desired

Conditions using this modification:

Inclusion: Diabetes mellitus, constipation, diverticular disease, general diet, high fiber diet, high potassium diet, low fat/cholesterol diet, reduced caloric/reduction diet

Exclusion: Gastrointestinal inflammatory diseases, diarrhea, clear liquid diets, low residue/bland/blenderized diet, mechanical soft except for soft fruits and juices, potassium restricted diet

Milk Exchanges:

12 g carbohydrate, 8 g protein, trace to 8 g fat, 90-150 calories per exchange depending on type of milk

Nonfat Milk:

Skim or nonfat milk	1 cup
Powdered nonfat milk	1/3 cup
Canned evaporated skim milk	1/2 cup
Buttermilk from skim milk	1 cup
Yogurt from skim milk (plain)	1 cup

Low Fat Milk:

1% or 2% fortified milk	1 cup
Yogurt from 2% milk	1 cup

Whole Milk:

4% whole milk	1 cup
Canned evaporated milk	1/2 cup
Buttermilk or yogurt (plain) from whole milk	1 cup

Conditions Using this Modification:

Inclusion: Diabetes mellitus, malnutrition, oral deterioration and disorders, high protein/high caloric diet, blenderized diet, low residue/bland diet, mechanical soft/pureed diet, general diet

Exclusion: Chronic renal failure, atherosclerosis, protein restricted diet, low fat/cholesterol diet, reduced caloric/reduction diet, clear liquid diet

Vegetable Exchanges:

5 g carbohydrate, 2 g protein, 25 calories/exchange

Asparagus	1/2 cup
Bean sprouts	1/2 cup
Beets	1/2 cup
Broccoli	1/2 cup
Cabbage, brussel sprouts	1/2 cup
Carrots	1/2 cup
Cauliflower	1/2 cup
Celery	1/2 cup
Eggplant	1/2 cup
Green pepper	1/2 cup
Beet, chard, collard, kale, mustard, spinach, turnip, dandelion greens	1/2 cup
Mushrooms	1/2 cup
Onions	1/2 cup
Okra, rutabaga, zucchini	1/2 cup
Sauerkraut	1/2 cup
Green, yellow beans	1/2 cup

Raw vegetables used as desired (lettuce, endive, escarole, parsley, watercress, radishes, chinese cabbage, cucumber)

Conditions using this modification:

Inclusion: Diabetes mellitus, constipation, diverticular disease, general diet, high fiber diet, high potassium diet, low fat/cholesterol diet, reduced caloric/reduction diet

Exclusion: Bowel inflammatory disease, oral deterioration and disorders, diarrhea, clear liquid diet blenderized, low residue/bland diet, mechanical soft diet unless pureed, potassium restricted diet

Meat Exchanges:

Lean Meats:

7 g protein, 3 g fat, 55 calories/exchange

Beef (baby beef, chuck, flank, tenderloin, round, tripe, ribs, rump)	1 oz
Lamb (leg, rib, sirloin, chops, roast, shank, shoulder)	1 oz
Pork (rump, shank, chops, ham)	1 oz
Veal (loin, rib, cutlets, shoulder, chops)	1 oz
Poultry (chicken, turkey, pheasant, without skin)	1 oz
Fish (fresh or frozen)	1 oz
Canned tuna, salmon, crab, lobster	1/4 cup
Shrimp, scallops, clams, oysters	1 oz
Sardines, drained	3
Cottage cheese (dry or 2%)	1/4 cup
Dried beans or peas (count as 1 meat and 1 starch)	1/2 cup
Cheese with less than 5% butterfat	1 oz

Medium Fat Meats:

7 g protein, 5 g fat, 75 calories/exchange

Beef (ground [15% fat round]), canned corned beef, rib eye roast or steak	1 oz
Pork (loin, tenderloin, shoulder arm or blade, broiled, ham, Canadian bacon)	1 oz
Liver, heart, kidney, sweetbreads	1 oz
Cottage cheese, creamed	1/4 cup

Cheese (ricotta, farmer's, parmesan, mozzarella)	1 oz
Egg	1
Peanut butter	2 tbsp

High Fat Meats:

7 g protein, 8 g fat, 100 calories/exchange

Beef (brisket, corned beef, ground chuck, roasts, steaks)	1 oz
Lamb breast, veal breast	1 oz
Pork (spare ribs, loin, ground, country ham)	1 oz
Poultry (capon, duck, goose)	1 oz
Cheese (cheddar)	1 oz
Cold cuts	1 slice
Frankfurter	1 small

Conditions using this modification:

Inclusion: Diabetes mellitus, anemia, all conditions with adjustments made for oral disorders, general diet, high protein/caloric diet, iron rich diet

Exclusion: Chronic renal failure, atherosclerosis, clear liquid and blenderized diets, mechanical soft/low residue/bland diets unless meat is pureed, low protein/reduced caloric diet, low fat/cholesterol, sodium diets unless modified

Fat Exchanges

Polyunsaturated

5 g fat, 45 calories/exchange

Margarine (corn, soy, safflower, cottonseed, sunflower)	1 tsp
Oil (corn, olive, peanut, soy, sunflower, safflower)	1 tsp
Avocado	1/8
Olives	8 large
Pecans	2 large
Walnuts	6 small
Almonds	6 whole
Spanish peanuts	20 whole
Virginia peanuts	10 whole

Saturated

Margarine (regular)	1 tsp
Butter	1 tsp
Light cream	1 tbsp
Sour cream	1 tbsp
Heavy cream	1 tbsp
Bacon fat	1 tsp
Bacon, crisp	1 strip
French, Italian dressing	1 tbsp
Mayonnaise	1 tsp
Mayonnaise-type salad dressing	2 tsp
Lard	1 tsp
Salt pork	3/4 in cube

Conditions using this modification:

Inclusion: Diabetes mellitus, general diet, high caloric diet

Exclusion: Reduced caloric diet, low fat/cholesterol diet, obesity, hypertension, coronary heart disease, atherosclerosis, cholecystitis/cholelithiasis, absorption disorders

Cultural/Ethnic Aspects of Exchanges

Cultural differences among older adults affect choices made regarding health care and food patterns in particular. The belief that a food is good or bad, and the influence of ethnicity on food selection affects eating patterns and nutritional status. The following lists include a limited selection of cultural/ethnic preferences, although many other foods are acceptable to these groups, especially if they are American born and have become acculturated. The lists are not complete, and menu planning should be based on nutritional assessment and exchanges made according to likes and dislikes.

Mexican American Selections:

Dairy products:	Custard (flan), Monterey jack cheese, rice pudding, milk with chocolate
Fruits, vegetables:	Corn, carrots, chili peppers, tomatoes, prickly pear cactus leaf and fruit, wild greens, shredded lettuce, melons, zapote, avocado
Meat, fish, eggs, legumes, nuts:	Pork and pork intestine, goat, tripe, sausage, pinto, garbanzo, calico, and refried beans, peanuts, eggs
Bread, cereals, grains, pasta, rice:	Tortillas, rice, pasta, sweet bread, cornmeal, polvillo, sopapilla
Supplementary:	Salt pork, tequila, lard, guacamole, chili sauce, chili powder, salsa, coriander, cumin, saffron, cinnamon, cocoa powder

African American Selections:

Dairy products:	Whole, dry, or evaporated milk, cottage and cheddar cheese
Fruits, vegetables:	Collard, kale, turnip and mustard greens, okra, beans, onions, sweet potatoes, yams, melons, tangerines

Meat, fish, eggs, legumes, nuts:	Pork and ham, hog jowls, ham hocks, hog maw, fatback, bacon, sausage, heart, lungs, kidneys, brains, pig's feet, tails, ears, and snout, neck bones, tongue, spareribs, squirrel, rabbit, opossum, quail, catfish, perch, salted fish, sardines, scallops, crayfish, black-eyed peas, peanuts, pinto and red kidney beans
Bread, cereals, grains, pasta, rice:	Hominy grits, biscuits, cornbread, hush puppies, spoon bread, baked sweet desserts
Supplementary:	Lard, gravies, molasses, syrups, jams and jellies

Asian Selections:

Dairy products:	Milk, cheese
Fruits, vegetables:	Bamboo shoots, green and yellow beans, bean sprouts, bok choy, eggplant, kale, collard, mustard, radish greens, leeks, mushrooms, peppers, scallions, snow peas, taro, tomatoes, water chestnuts, white radishes, dates, figs, grapes, kumquats, litchee nuts, mangoes, papayas, persimmons, napa cabbage, seaweed, limes, cherries, pomegranates, pickled plums, tangerines
Meat, fish, eggs, legumes, nuts:	Pork, beef, organ meats, goat, duck, carp, oysters, lobster, crab, mackerel, sardines, abalone, eel, squid, octopus, fish sausage, globefish, sushi, soybean curd, soybean paste, soybeans, lima and red beans, chestnuts, almonds, cashews
Bread, cereals, grains, pasta, rice:	Rice, noodles, barley, millet, lemon grass, oatmeal, fortune cookie, cellophane noodles

Supplementary:	Soy sauce, sweet and sour sauce, ginger, pickled vegetables, suet, saki, plum sauce, peanut oil, lard, mustard sauce

Italian Selections:

Dairy products:	Milk, parmesan, ricotta, romano, provolone, and other cheeses, custard
Fruits, vegetables:	Escarole, zucchini, squashes, eggplant, artichokes, peppers, tomatoes, swiss chard, dandelion and mustard greens, fennel, tangerines, figs, persimmons, pomegranates, olives, melons, quinces, dates
Meat, fish, eggs, legumes, nuts:	Beef, veal, organ meats, lamb, pork, salami, peppered sausage, prosciutto, sardines, anchovies, shell fish, octopus, snails, squid, chick peas, lentils, almonds, pistachios, walnuts, chestnuts
Bread, cereals, grains, pasta, rice:	White Italian bread, all pasta products, pizza grains, pasta, rice, corn meal, polenta
Supplementary:	Olive oil, garlic, vinegar, oregano, basil, saffron, parsley, salt pork, espresso, lard, chianti wine

Mideastern Selections:

Dairy products:	Soured milk (cow, goat, sheep), soft and hard cheeses (feta), yogurt
Fruits, vegetables:	Onions, tomatoes, okra, peppers, eggplant, cucumber, grape leaves, artichoke, cabbage, leeks, greens, olives, melons, dates, figs, grapes, quinces, apricots, plums, currants, raisins, prunes, cherries, oranges

Meat, fish, eggs, legumes, nuts:	Mutton, lamb, goat, beef, pork, camel, goose, duck, salted and smoked fish, eggs, lentils, chick peas, soybeans, peanuts, pistachios, caraway and sesame seeds, hummus
Bread, cereals, grains, pasta, rice:	Dark and whole cracked wheat bread, rice, barley, pita bread, corn, baklava pastry, couscous
Supplementary:	Meat fats, olive and seed oils, honey, lemon juice, sour cream, turkish coffee and paste, apricot candy

Jewish Selections:

Dairy products:	Milk, buttermilk, almost all cheeses, especially cottage and cream cheese, sour cream
Fruits, vegetables:	All vegetables, shav, potato latkes, borscht, all fruits with preference for dried fruits, oranges, apricots, apples
Meat, fish, eggs, legumes, nuts:	Kosher beef, lamb, veal, chicken, goose, turkey, duck, pigeon, carp, whitefish, caviar, smoked or salted fish, gefilte fish, lentils, dried beans, delicatessen corned beef, hot dogs, pastrami, and salami, chopped liver
Bread, cereals, grains, pasta, rice:	Brown and white rice, rye, pumpernickel breads, rolls with seeds, challah bread, matzo, farfel, kasha or greats, bagels, blintzes, bialys, matzo balls, strudel, cheesecake, macaroons, sponge cake
Supplementary:	Butter, shmaltz (chicken fat), vegetable oil, wine, kosher pickles, preserves

Vegetarian Selections:

Dairy products:	All milks, cheeses, ice cream, yogurt
Fruits, vegetables:	All fresh, canned, frozen dried fruits and vegetables, fruit and vegetable juices
Meat, fish, eggs, legumes, nuts:	No meat or poultry; allowed are eggs, nuts, legumes (especially soybeans); some allow fish
Bread, cereals, grains, pasta, rice:	All breads with emphasis on whole wheat types, whole grain cereals, rice, all pasta
Supplementary:	Avoid fats, sweets; other supplements and condiments allowed

Chapter VII

DIET THERAPY/EXCHANGE LISTS FOR COMMON DISORDERS

A. Hematologic Disorders
    Anemia
B. Cardiovascular Disorders
    Coronary Artery Disease
    Hypertension
C. Endocrine Disorders
    Diabetes Mellitus
D. Gastrointestinal/Hepatic/Biliary Disorders
    Diverticular Disease
    Inflammatory/Irritable Bowel Disease
    Gallbladder Disease
E. Musculoskeletal Disorders
    Osteoporosis
    Arthritis
F. Renal Disorders
    Chronic Renal Failure
G. Other Disorders
    Malnutrition
    Constipation
    Diarrhea
    Fluid/Electrolyte Imbalance
    Nausea
    Oral Mucositis/Stomatitis
    Wound Healing

Hematologic Disorders

Anemia

General Information:

Anemia is a condition resulting from a decrease in the number of red blood cells (RBC) or changes in the structure or function of these cells. One type commonly affecting the older adult is nutritional anemia, caused by a dietary deficiency of iron or folic acid (iron or folate deficiency anemia), or deficiency of B_{12} as a result of an absence of intrinsic factor (pernicious anemia). A second type is associated with chronic diseases such as inflammatory bowel disease, arthritis, renal disease, and infections that involve various other nutrients, or persistent or chronic gastrointestinal blood loss. Signs and symptoms of anemia vary with the severity of the disorder, and relate to the body's response to hypoxia, since the function of the RBCs is to carry oxygen to all body organs and tissues.

Mild anemia (hemoglobin of 10-14 g/dL) doesn't usually produce symptoms except following strenuous activity (palpitations, dyspnea, dizziness). Moderate anemic states (hemoglobin of 6-10 g/dL) produce the same symptoms with the addition of diaphoresis and fatigue, both during rest and activity. Severe anemia (hemoglobin of <6 g/dL) produces a multisystem response of pallor, jaundice, pruritus, dyspnea, tachypnea, orthopnea, sore mouth and tongue, palpitations, tachycardia, fatigue, weakness, nausea, headache, dizziness, irritability, malaise, as well as hematemesis, hematuria, and tarry feces in association with chronic blood loss. The most common causes of iron deficiency anemia in the older adult are inadequate nutritional intake, inadequate intestinal absorption of iron, and increased erythropoiesis as a result of chronic blood loss.

Management of iron or folic acid deficiency anemia involves the administration of iron preparations orally (ferrous sulfate) or intramuscularly (iron dextran), or folic acid orally, or by dietary inclusions. Treatment for pernicious anemia involves the intramuscular administration of vitamin B_{12} (cyanocobalamin) for life and supplemental intake or dietary inclusions of the vitamin. Diagnostic test and procedure considerations include complete blood count (CBC) with emphasis on RBC, RBC indices, Hb, Hct, serum iron, iron-combining capacity, serum folate, serum ferritin, gastrointestinal tract radiology series, and Schillings test.

Dietary Implications:

Include foods high in protein, iron, folate, and vitamins in the diet

Avoid overcooking, which destroys essential nutrients

Select foods that allow for cultural/ethnic preferences when possible

Exchange Lists for Foods High in Iron/Folic Acid/B$_{12}$

Iron	Folic Acid	Vitamin B$_{12}$
Bread/Cereal:		
Oatmeal	Whole grains in bread or cereals	
Bran flakes	Wheat germ	
White enriched/ whole wheat bread	Enriched breads, flour products	
Pasta		
Dairy Products:		
Egg yolk	Yogurt, eggs	Milk, yogurt
Meat:		
Liver, liverwurst; beef, beef patty; fish/shrimp; chicken, lamb, pork; frankfurter	Liver; fish (cod)	Organ/muscle meats; clams, salmon

Vegetable:

Spinach/dark green leafy vegetables	Green leafy vegetables
Peas, snap beans	Asparagus, potato
Split peas/legumes	
Potato	

Fruit:

Dried fruits (prunes, raisins, figs)	Nuts Orange juice
Orange, peach	Banana Cantaloupe
Grapes, cherries	Lemon, strawberries

Cardiovascular Disorders

Coronary Artery Disease

General Information:

Coronary artery disease is a condition resulting from athero-sclerosis (deposits of lipid materials on the intima of vessels) of the arteries of the heart causing narrowing of the vessels and a potential for reduced blood flow to the heart muscle. Atherosclerosis is common in older adults, although some are more at risk for developing this condition than others. It is the main cause of heart diseases such as angina and myocardial infarction, and cerebral infarction (stroke). Risk factors associated with this condition are being overweight with a high intake of calories, high intake of fats and cholesterol, sedentary lifestyle, smoking, age, and stress.

Management involves following a low fat/cholesterol diet to treat hyperlipidemia, consisting of no more than 30% calories from fat/day, no more than 10% saturated fat/day, and 250-300 mg cholesterol/day. Low caloric/reduction diets and daily exercise routines to improve circulation and control weight

are also emphasized. Lipid lowering agents may be administered. Diagnostic procedure and test considerations include
coronary angiography, exercise stress testing, nuclear scanning,
and lipid panel (cholesterol, triglycerides, low density lipids
[LDL], high density lipids [HDL]).

Dietary Implications:

Low fat/cholesterol food inclusion can also provide low
caloric intake for weight reduction goal

Exchange Lists for Foods Low in
Fat/Cholesterol and Calories

Low Fat/Cholesterol

See Gallbladder Disease for low
fat/cholesterol inclusions
for exchanges

Low Caloric/Reduction

See Gallbladder Disease for low
caloric/reduction inclusions for
exchanges

Hypertension

General Information:

Hypertension is generally defined as a systolic blood pressure
of 140 mmHg and diastolic blood pressure of 90 mmHg or
more. The condition can be classified as systolic or diastolic,
or primary or secondary hypertension. The most common
condition is primary (essential) hypertension that develops
from factors such as an increase in cardiac output or peripheral
resistance. These factors are affected by renal regulation of
sodium, arteriosclerosis, and loss of elastic tissue in large
vessels associated with aging. In the older adult, the most
common types are isolated systolic (a systolic reading of 160
with a normal or slightly increased diastolic reading) and the
combined systolic-diastolic (an increased systolic and diastolic
reading). Risk factors for developing the disease include age,
sex, ethnicity, stress, obesity, alcoholism, smoking, and dietary
intake of sodium.

Management involves dietary modifications of sodium (1-2.5 g/day or 4-6 g sodium chloride/day), fat/cholesterol restrictions, low caloric/reduction to control weight if needed, and high potassium dietary intake, especially if on diuretic therapy. A planned daily exercise routine is also advised to maintain weight loss. Medication regimens include antihypertensive agents and diuretics. Diagnostic test considerations include urinalysis, serum sodium and potassium, lipid panel (cholesterol, triglycerides, low and high density lipids), glucose, creatinine, and BUN.

Dietary Implications:

Alcohol intake should be limited to < 2 ounces/day

Potassium, calcium, magnesium can be included in management and supplied in foods or oral supplements

Salt is not used in food preparation and salt shaker is removed from the tray

Foods high in potassium may contain sodium and need to be regulated to conform to sodium restriction

Exchange Lists of Foods Low in Fat/Cholesterol, Sodium, Calories and High Potassium Diets

High Potassium	Low Fat/Cholesterol, Caloric/Reduction, Sodium
Bread/Cereal:	
Whole grain breads, bran cereals	See Gallbladder Disease for low fat/cholesterol inclusions for exchanges
Meat:	
All meats and poultry	See Fluid/Electrolyte Imbalance for low sodium inclusions for exchanges

Vegetable:

Broccoli, potatoes, legumes, brussel sprouts, parsnips, pumpkin, winter squash; tomato, tomato juice; vegetable juices

See Gallbladder Disease for low caloric/reduction inclusions for exchanges

Fruit:

Bananas, papaya, melons; all citrus fruits and juices; dried dates, raisins, prunes, and other fruits; avocado, rhubarb

Miscellaneous:

Pecans, walnuts, peanuts; broth, bouillon; chocolate, cocoa, molasses; eggs; coffee, tea, salt substitute

Endocrine Disorders

Diabetes Mellitus

General Information:

Older adults develop a decrease in the ability to metabolize glucose. Type 2 or adult onset diabetes mellitus is a common disease among the older adult population. This age group is more apt to develop degenerative changes and complications that require hospitalization as a result of diabetes. Type 1 diabetes mellitus is a second type that can be present in the older adult, but is not as common. Risk factors for Type 2 include familial tendency, obesity (requires more insulin for the amount of food eaten), and age (reduced pancreatic function).

Management involves dietary modifications that include a balanced diet with food selections and amounts that meet caloric requirements and offer exchanges or substitutes to control blood glucose levels. Dietary inclusions for meal planning are available from the American Dietetic Association. Dietary intake is planned in conjunction with the administration of insulin SC or hypoglycemics orally (depending on the type of diabetes) and planned daily exercises or activities. Diagnostic tests include blood glucose, glycosylated hemoglobin, and urinary glucose and ketones.

Dietary Implications:

Eat all of the food allowed on the diet, eat meals and snacks at the suggested times, never omit a meal, eat foods in correct portions stated on exchange lists

Use noncaloric artificial sweeteners and fat substitutes in foods and beverages

Limit alcohol intake to < 2 ounces/day to be taken with meals

Avoid the addition of sugar to foods and beverages or foods sweetened with sugar or honey; avoid saturated fat selections in diet

Exchange Lists for Diabetic Diet*

Starch/Bread Group:

Each exchange contains carbohydrate (15 g), protein (3 g), and fat (trace) that totals 80 calories; 1/2 cup of cereals/pasta or 1 oz of bread can be used for servings of foods on or off the list.

Flaked bran cereals	1/2 cup	Bagel	1/2
Cooked cereals	1/2 cup	English muffin	1/2
Other unsweetened cereals	3/4 cup	Small roll	1 oz
Whole wheat, rye, and white bread	1 slice	Puffed cereals	1 1/2 cup
Shredded wheat	1/2 cup	Tortilla	1

White or brown rice	1/3 cup	Pita	1/2
Pasta	1/2 cup	Hamburger/ hot dog bun	1/2
Dried beans/peas/ lentils	1/2 cup	Baked beans	1/3 cup
Crackers	6	Lima beans/ peas	2/3 cup 1/2 cup
Graham crackers	3	Small baked potato	1
Melba toast	5	Mashed potato	1/2 cup
Popcorn	3 cups	Corn	1/2 cup
Pretzels	3/4 oz	Small baked potato	1
Rye Crisp	4	Squash	3/4 cup
Matzo	3/4 oz	Yam, sweet potato	1/2 cup
Whole wheat crackers	2-4 slices		

Meat Group:

Each exchange contains carbohydrate in lean or fat meat (0 g), protein in lean or fat meat (7 g), and fat in lean (3 g) or medium fat (5 g) or high fat (8 g) meats that totals 55, 75, 100 calories respectively.

Lean		**Medium fat**		**High fat**	
Beef (round, sirloin, flank steak, tenderloin, chipped beef)	1 oz	Beef (ground, roasts, steak, meatloaf)	1 oz	Beef (ribs, corned beef)	1 oz

Lean		Medium fat		High fat	
Pork (fresh ham, boiled ham, Canadian bacon, tenderloin)	1 oz	Pork (chops, loin roast, cutlets, butt roast)	1 oz	Pork (spareribs, ground, pork sausage)	1 oz
Veal (chops, roast)	1 oz	Veal cutlet	1 oz		
Poultry without skin	1 oz	Poultry with skin	1 oz		
Venison, rabbit	1 oz	Lamb (roast, chops)	1 oz	Lamb patty	1 oz
Fish (all fresh/ frozen)	1 oz	Fish (canned tuna, salmon drained)	1/4 cup	Fish (fried)	1 oz
Fresh or canned lobster, crab, shrimp, clams	2 oz				
Oysters	6				
Tuna, water packed	1/4 cup				
Herring	1 oz				

Lean		Medium fat		High fat	
Canned sardines	2				
Cheese, cottage	1/4 cup	Skim milk, cheeses	1/4 cup	All cheeses	1 oz
Diet cheeses	1 oz	Diet cheeses	1 oz		
Grated parmesan	2 tbsp				
Fat free lunch meat (95%)	1 oz	Fat free lunch meat (86%)	1 oz	All lunch meat; sausages	1 oz
Egg whites	3	Egg substitute	1/4 cup	Frank-furter	1
Egg substitute	1/4 cup	Tofu	4 oz	Peanut butter	1 tbsp

Vegetable Group:

Each exchange contains carbohydrate (5 g), protein (2 g), fat (0 g) that totals 25 calories; 1/2 cup of cooked vegetables or 1 cup of raw vegetables can be used for each serving on or off the list. Starchy vegetables are included in the Starch/Bread list.

Artichoke (1/2)	Asparagus	Green, wax beans
Bean sprouts	Beets	Broccoli
Brussel sprouts	Cabbage	Carrots
Cauliflower	Eggplant	Collard, mustard, turnip greens
Kohlrabi	Leek	Mushrooms
Okra	Onions	Green peppers
Rutabaga	Sauerkraut	Spinach
Summer squash	Tomato	Turnips
Zucchini	Vegetable juice	

Fruit Group:

Each exchange contains carbohydrate (15 g) that totals 60 calories; 1/2 cup of fresh fruit or juice or 1/4 cup of dried fruit can be used for each serving on or off the list.

Fresh, frozen, or unsweetened canned fruits		Dried fruit		Fruit juice	
Apple	1	Apples	4 pieces	Apple cider/juice	1/2 cup
Applesauce	1/2 cup	Apricots	7	Cranberry juice	1/3 cup
Apricots	4 raw/ 1/2 cup	Dates	3	Grapefruit juice	1/2 cup
Banana	1 small	Figs	2 medium	Grape juice	1/3 cup
Black-/ Blue-berries	3/4 cup	Prunes	3	Orange juice	1/2 cup
Cherries	12 raw/ 1/2 cup	Raisins	2 tbsp	Pineapple juice	1/2 cup
Cantaloupe	1/3 melon			Prune juice	1/3 cup
Fruit cocktail	1/2 cup				
Grapefruit	1/2				
Grapefruit segment	3/4 cup				
Grapes	17 small				
Honeydew	1 cup cubes				
Nectarine	1				

Fruit Group:

Orange	1
Peach, pear	1
Peach, pear canned	1/2 cup
Pineapple	3/4 cup
Pineapple, canned	1/3 cup
Plum	2
Rasp-berries	1 cup
Straw-berries	1 1/4 cup
Tangerine	2
Water-melon	1 1/4 cup

Milk Group:

Each exchange contains carbohydrate (12 g), protein (8 g), and fat in very low fat (trace), low fat (5 g), and whole (8 g) that totals 90, 120, 150 calories respectively.

Very low fat		Low Fat		Whole	
Skim milk	1 cup	2% milk	1 cup	Whole milk	1 cup
1/2% milk	1 cup	Plain yogurt	8 oz	Evaporated	1/2 cup
1% milk	1 cup				
Low fat buttermilk	1 cup			Whole plain yogurt	1/2 cup

Very low fat		Low Fat		Whole	
Dry nonfat milk	1/3 cup				
Plain nonfat yogurt	8 oz				
Evaporated skim milk	1/2 cup				

Fat Group:

Each exchange contains 5 gm fat and 45 calories

Unsaturated fats:

Avocado	1/8	Cottonseed, corn, safflower, soybean, olive, peanut oils	1 tsp
Margarine, diet	1 tbsp	Olives	10 large
Mayonnaise, diet	1 tbsp	Salad dressing, mayonnaise type	2 tsp
Almonds, dry roasted	6	Salad dressing all others	1 tbsp
Pecans	2 whole		
Peanuts	10 nuts		
Walnuts	2		
Seeds	1 tbsp		

Free group:

All salad greens	1/2 cup	Drinks (broth, bouillon, coffee, tea, sugar free carbonated drinks and water, sugar free drink mix)
Cranberries, rhubarb	1/2 cup	
Raw vegetables (celery, cabbage, cucumber, onion, peppers, radishes, zucchini)		

Catsup,	1 Tbsp	Sugar	2 Tbsp
taco sauce,		substitutes	
horseradish,		Whipped	
mustard,		topping	
pickles, vinegar			
		Sodium free	
		seasonings and	
		soy sauce,	
		lemon, lime	
		juices	

Modified from The American Diabetes Association and The American Dietetic Association, Exchange Lists for Meal Planning, 1995.

Gastrointestinal/Hepatic/Biliary Disorders

Diverticular Disease

General Information:

Diverticulosis is a common disease in the older adult. It is characterized by the formation of pouches in the wall of the colon and can cause abdominal pain and alternate diarrhea and constipation patterns. It is thought to be caused by dietary intake deficient in fiber and bulk, causing an increase in intraluminal pressure in a colon that has lost elasticity with aging.

Management related to nutrition includes a diet high in fiber as tolerated, a low to moderate residue diet, or a minimum residue diet depending on the acuteness of the condition and what is most beneficial to the individual. Diagnostic procedure consideration includes barium enema radiologic examination and colonoscopy.

Dietary Implications:

Avoid nuts, seeds, raw fruits and vegetables, and fried foods in high fiber diet

Low residue/bland diet should be given for diverticulitis

Exchange Lists for Foods High in Fiber and Low Residue/Bland

High Fiber

See Constipation for high fiber inclusions for exchanges

Low Residue/Bland and Modified Bland

See Diarrhea for low residue/bland inclusions for exchanges

Modified Bland:

Bread/Cereal: White, whole wheat, rye bread made with refined wheat without seeds or raisins; crackers, rolls, biscuits, toast; cooked and ready to eat cereal from refined grains, oatmeal; white rice, plain pasta

Dairy Products: Whole, skim milk, buttermilk, yogurt, sour cream, butter, eggs, cottage cheese, other processed cheeses

Meat: Tender beef, veal, ham, liver, fish, shellfish (broiled, baked, stewed); canned tuna or salmon

Vegetable: White or sweet potatoes without skin (baked, mashed, boiled); well cooked or canned vegetables; chopped raw vegetables

Fruit: All fruit juices, ripe fresh fruits that are peeled without seeds; frozen or canned fruits; melons, citrus fruit segments

Dessert: Plain pie, cake, cookies, pudding, ice cream, sherbet, gelatin

Miscellaneous: Finely chopped spices and herbs; soy sauce, vinegar, salt, catsup, chocolate, sauces, gravies, broth- and cream-based soups; coffee, tea, carbonated beverages, cereal beverages

Inflammatory/Irritable Bowel Disease

General Information:

Gastroenteritis is an inflammatory condition of the stomach and intestinal tract and causes abdominal cramping, nausea, vomiting, and diarrhea. It can be caused by viral or bacterial microorganisms and can be serious in the older debilitated adult. Irritable bowel syndrome (spastic colon) is a dysfunctional condition (motility changes) of the small and large intestine causing abdominal pain, anorexia, nausea, and constipation or diarrhea. It is thought to be caused by stress, and dietary intake of low residue, high fat, and gas producing foods.

Management for gastroenteritis involves resting the bowel, providing a clear fluid diet, increasing fluid intake during acute stages, and administration of antispasmodics and anti-diarrheals. Management for irritable bowel involves dietary inclusion of fiber to treat constipation and diarrhea, and administration of anti-anxiety agents during stressful episodes. Diagnostic test considerations include fecal examination for abnormal constituents and microorganism identification.

Dietary Implications:

Avoid food inclusions that are gas forming or irritating such as beans, milk and milk products, alcohol, and caffeinated beverages

Exchange Lists for Foods High in Fiber and Low Residue/Bland Diet

High Fiber

See Constipation for inclusions for exchanges

Low Residue/Bland

See Diverticular Disease for inclusions for exchanges

Gallbladder Disease

General Information:

Gallbladder disease in the older adult includes chronic or acute cholecystitis (inflammation) and cholelithiasis (gallstones) with possible symptoms of pain, nausea, vomiting, and jaundice. The presence of cholelithiasis in the older adult can cause shakiness and changes in mentation rather than the usual symptoms. Cholesterol saturation of the bile increases with age and contributes to gallbladder abnormalities (changes in the bile composition and bile stasis). Obesity is also a risk factor associated with gallbladder disease. Treatment depends upon the severity of symptoms and can lead to cholecystectomy or possibly percutaneous cholecystolithotomy. Drugs to reduce cholesterol in the bile can also be administered.

Management involves a reduction/low caloric diet in combination with supplemental vitamins and minerals if overweight, and maintenance of a low fat/cholesterol diet. Diagnostic procedures and tests include ultrasound, computerized tomography, oral or intravenous cholecystography, and bilirubin if obstruction is present.

Dietary Implications

Include a daily exercise routine for successful weight loss and maintenance

Reduce the size of servings and eliminate between meal snacks in low caloric dietary regimen

Low fat dietary intake decreases gallbladder contractions

Fat should not be added when preparing foods

Seasonings can replace fats to add flavor to the diet

Exchange Lists for Foods Low in Fat/Cholesterol, Calories

Low Fat/Cholesterol

Bread/Cereal:

Enriched white and whole grain breads; English muffins, melba toast; low fat white crackers, graham crackers; hot breads, pancakes, waffles made with substitute egg; all cereals except granola, or those with coconut or high fat content; pasta products made without egg

Dairy Products:

Skim milk, buttermilk; cottage cheese, cheeses with less than 11% fat; egg white, cholesterol free egg substitute; margarine

Meat:

Lean or fat trimmed beef, veal, pork, lamb; poultry with skin removed; low fat cold cuts; canned tuna or salmon in water; fish, clams, scallops, lobster, oysters; broth-based canned or homemade soups

Reduction/Low Caloric

Limited amount of whole wheat or English muffin, melba toast, 3-4 low fat crackers (any variety); limited amount of pancakes or waffles, rolls or bran muffins; all low caloric dry/cooked cereals; pasta products

Skim milk; low fat cottage cheese; egg; limited amount of margarine

Lean beef, veal, pork, lamb, poultry; low fat cold cuts; canned tuna or salmon in water; all seafood (baked or steamed); beef or chicken broth

Vegetable:

All vegetables prepared without butter or cream sauces; all vegetable juices; vegetable oils (corn, soy, cottonseed, safflower, peanut)

All raw and cooked vegetables (plain); all vegetable juices

Fruit:

All fresh/canned fruits and fruit juices

All fresh fruits and fruit juices; sugar free canned fruit

Dessert:

Gelatin, ices, low fat frozen desserts, sherbet; angel food cake, ginger snaps, vanilla wafers; pudding made with skim milk

Sugar free gelatin; sugar free custard made with skim milk

Miscellaneous:

Peanut butter, nuts, olives (limited); mustard, catsup, steak sauces, gravies made with fat free broth; hard candies, syrups, honey, jellies, jams, marshmallows; salad dressings (commercial or homemade), cholesterol free or made with unsaturated fat; carbonated beverages, cocoa made with skim milk

Peanut butter; condiments; sugar free beverages; sugar free candy; low calorie salad dressings, jellies

Musculoskeletal Disorders

Osteoporosis

General Information:

Osteoporosis is a metabolic bone disease in the older adult associated with a reduction in bone mass resulting from a faster rate of bone reabsorption than bone formation. As bone mineral and matrix is decreased, bone fracture, bone pain, spinal deformity (widow's hump), and a loss in height can occur. The primary type is related to postmenopausal status and the secondary type is related to an underlying condition such as hyperparathyroidism, hyperthyroidism, or long-term steroid therapy. Included in the primary type is the postmenopausal (ages 50-75) and senile (age 70 or more) osteoporosis affecting females two times more than males.

Management of osteoporosis involves prevention by use of oral or dietary supplements of calcium (700-1,500 mg/day) and vitamin D, treatment with estrogen replacement or calcitonin therapy, and possibly fluoride treatment. A planned daily exercise routine is also important to prevent the loss of minerals from the bones. Diagnostic tests known as densitometry or x-ray absorptiometry are available to measure bone mass in the body.

Dietary Implications:

Vitamin D fortified foods should be included in the diet high in calcium

Protein, sodium, and fiber inclusions in the diet are necessary to reduce calcium loss

Avoid alcohol and tobacco use, both of which have an effect on bones if calcium intake is deficient

Exchange List for Foods High in Calcium

Dairy Products:

Whole, skim milk (fortified with vitamin D)

Buttermilk, eggnog, half and half

Evaporated canned milk

Ice cream, yogurt, custard

Cheddar, creamed cottage,
American, mozzarella, Swiss,
parmesan cheeses

Calcium fortified soy milk

Seafood:

Sardines, shrimp, salmon, oysters

Vegetable:

Spinach, broccoli, collard, turnip,
and mustard greens

Bok choy, kale

Bean curd (tofu)

Fruit:

Orange juice fortified with calcium

Nuts:

Almonds, hazelnuts

Arthritis

General Information:

The most common arthritis found in the older adult is osteo-
arthritis, although rheumatoid arthritis with onset in middle
age continues to cause health problems in the older adult.
Both types result in inflammation in the joints and pain that
affects movement and activity. Nonsteroidal anti-inflammatory
analgesics are usually prescribed for pain control.

Management associated with nutrition includes a low caloric/
reduction diet to relieve stress on damaged or deteriorated
joints caused by excessive body weight. Diagnostic procedure
considerations include radiologic x-ray of involved joints.

Dietary Implications:

Food selections for those with rheumatoid arthritis
should avoid food allergies or intolerances

A daily exercise routine combined with a reduction diet
for successful weight control can be modified to meet
individual mobility and movement abilities

See Gallbladder Disease for
all foods allowed with exchanges
for low caloric, low fat foods in
each group

Food servings reduced to meet
1,000-1,600 kcal/day as prescribed

Renal Disorders

Chronic Renal Failure

General Information:

Chronic renal failure (CRF) is a progressive disease characterized by the destruction of kidney tissue resulting in impaired function. It is most commonly caused by hypertension and diabetes mellitus. A person suffering from CRF is also predisposed to other kidney diseases. CRF is associated with regulatory problems of fluid and electrolyte balance (potassium, sodium, calcium, phosphate), and changes affecting protein, carbohydrate, and fat metabolism. Fluid balance is more difficult to maintain in the older adult due to the number of nephrons being greatly reduced, and the likelihood of pre-existing conditions being present.

Management involves fluid and dietary protein restrictions, potassium and sodium dietary restrictions, and dialysis therapy, all dependent on glomerular filtration rate (GFR). A GFR of 6 mL/minute is managed with a dietary protein restriction of 40 g/day that usually also contains about 2.8 g/day of potassium. Sodium is usually restricted to 1-3 g/day and fluids to 1,500-3,000 mL/day or 400-500 mL + urinary output volume depending on sodium balance. Diagnostic procedure and test considerations include kidney, ureter, bladder radiologic x-ray, renal angiography, computerized scan, intravenous pyelogram, and electrolyte panel, BUN, CBC, urinalysis, creatinine clearance.

Dietary Implications:

Provide 35-45 kcal/kg/day of body weight with protein limited to 150-250 kcal/day; protein should be specifically prescribed as 20 g, 40 g, 60 g

Offer high calorie foods, and high caloric, low protein commercial supplements

Exchange Lists for Foods Low in Potassium, Sodium, Protein

Low Potassium	Low Protein	Low Sodium
Bread/Cereal:		
All breads and cereals; all pastas	All breads/cereals; all pastas	See Fluid/Electrolyte Imbalance for low sodium inclusions for exchanges
Dairy Products:		
Cottage cheese, eggs	Butter, sour cream	
Meat:		
Meats, chicken, fish	Limited amounts of meats and fish	
Vegetable:		
Lettuce, radishes, tomatoes, green peppers, green beans; vegetable oils; drained canned vegetables	Carrots, lettuce, onions, radishes, eggplant, squash, cabbage, cucumbers, tomatoes	
Fruit:		
Cranberry juice, lemons, blueberries; drained canned fruits	Apples, peaches, pears, berries, cherries, grapefruit, pineapple	

Miscellaneous:

| Tapioca; salad dressing; coffee, tea | Hard candies; coffee, tea; carbonated drinks |

Other Disorders

Malnutrition

General Information

Malnutrition is a condition characterized by overweight (20% more than desirable) with increases in body fat, or underweight (10% less than desirable) with losses in lean and fat body masses. Overweight problems in the older adult are generally caused by ingesting too many calorics (fattening foods) and alcoholic beverages, decreasing metabolism, and a sedentary lifestyle with little or no exercise due to energy and stamina decline. It can also result from psychiatric disorders or continuation of obesity from childhood. Underweight problems in the older adult are generally caused by decreased ingestion of food, selective pattern of ingesting the same limited foods every day, and the presence of chronic illness with anorexia, or changes in taste, chewing, and swallowing abilities common with the aging process. Weight loss in the older adult can indicate a pathologic process. Medication therapy can also influence weight gains and losses by stimulating or decreasing food intake and causing confusion and neglect in eating and drinking. Medications can also cause diarrhea, vomiting, and other excessive fluid losses and absorption problems affecting weight status.

Management includes dietary changes that involve reduced (1,000-1,200 kcal/day or 250-350 kcal/meal) or increased (1,800-2000 kcal/day) caloric content. An established exercise routine will also assist in weight control and preserve muscle mass.

Dietary Implications:

Supplemental foods and fluids can be offered between meals and at bedtime to increase caloric intake

Supplement powders can be added to liquids and solid foods to increase caloric intake

Dietary intake that is nutritionally adequate but higher in carbohydrate and lower in fat can result in caloric reduction

American Diabetes and Food Exchange System can be used to plan weight reduction diets

Exchange Lists for Low Caloric and High Caloric/Protein Diets

Low Caloric
(Amounts based on calories allowed for weight loss goal)

Bread/Cereal:

Enriched white/ whole grain breads

English muffins, melba toast

Pita bread, tortillas

Low fat crackers, graham, matzo, saltines

Hot breads, pancakes, waffles made with skim milk

All dry and cooked cereals

Limited pasta products

Dairy Products:

Skim milk, buttermilk, yogurt

Low fat cottage cheese, alpine lace cheese

Eggs

Margarine

High Caloric/Protein

See Wound Healing for high caloric/protein inclusions for exchanges

Meat:

Lean beef, pork, veal, lamb (all trimmed of fat before cooking)

Poultry with skin removed

Low fat dried cold cuts

Fish, clams, scallops, lobster, oysters

Water packed tuna, salmon, sardines

Broth-based canned or homemade soups

Vegetable:

All raw or cooked vegetables prepared without butter or cream sauces

Vegetable juices

Vegetable oils and salad dressings (low fat/caloric)

Fruit:

All raw fruits

Canned low caloric fruits

Dessert:

Gelatin/frozen desserts (low caloric), ices, sherbet

Angel food cake, vanilla wafers

Pudding made with skim milk

Miscellaneous:

Peanut butter

Mustard, catsup, steak sauces

Hard candy, syrup, honey, jellies
(low caloric)

Carbonated beverages, cocoa with
skim milk

Constipation

General Information:

Constipation is a condition or symptom resulting from decreased peristalsis, intestinal blockage caused by an abnormality such as a tumor, or inadequate intake of fluid or bulk foods. It can become a chronic condition in the older adult causing a decrease in the number of bowel movements and difficult passage of hard feces. Conditions that are associated with constipation include degenerative neurologic diseases such as Parkinson's and cerebrovascular accident, hypothyroidism, stress induced irritable bowel syndrome, spastic colon and dehydration. Chronic use of or dependence on laxatives, and administration of other medication regimens such as antacids, minerals (calcium, iron), narcotics, or anticholinergics can also contribute to the problem. The most common complication of constipation is fecal impaction.

For some older adults, constipation can exist for years. Management involves the increase of dietary fiber (25-35 g/day), increase of fluid intake (2,000 mL/day), and establishment of a daily exercise routine. Laxatives (bulk forming agent such as psyllium), suppositories, or enemas are only advocated when all other measures have been unsuccessful.

Dietary Implications:

Cook foods such as beans, peas, lentils into a soft soupy consistency for those with chewing or swallowing problems

Increase fluid intake, especially with fiber intake in those with dysphagia or esophageal problems to prevent obstruction in the esophagus

Add wheat, bran, or cereals to soups, chopped meats, vegetables, or casseroles for those who do not eat rolls, cookies, breads, or dry cereals

Exchange List for Foods High in Fiber/Bulk

Bread/Cereal:

Flour and bread (whole wheat, bran, white, cornmeal, buckwheat)

Cereals (All-Bran, Grapenuts, oatmeal, cornflakes, puffed rice or wheat, Rice Krispies, shredded wheat, Total, Wheaties)

Cookies and muffins (oatmeal, bran, dried fruit)

Rice (brown and white)

Vegetable:

Raw vegetables, lettuce, carrots, celery, spinach, cabbage, broccoli, asparagus, cauliflower, corn, peppers, beets, dried peas and beans, green beans

Fruit:

Dried fruits (apricots, figs, prunes, dates, pears, raisins)

Raw fruits with skins (apples, plums, peaches, grapes, pears, berries, cherries)

Peeled fruits (oranges, grapefruit, rhubarb)

Canned fruits (grapefruit, mandarin oranges, strawberries)

Nuts:

Peanuts, pecans, brazils, almonds

Popcorn, seeds

Diarrhea

General Information:

Diarrhea is a condition or symptom resulting from an increase in the movement of contents through the intestinal tract (peristalsis) caused by the stomach and intestinal attempt to eliminate any mucosal irritant. The most common causes in the older adult are diverticular disease (atrophy or weakness of the muscles of the bowel), irritable bowel (altered motility brought about by diet or stress), or infectious/inflammatory conditions (bacterial, stress or immunologic response). An alternate pattern of diarrhea and constipation can be produced by these abnormal bowel diseases. Nutritional and fluid deficiencies can develop with persistent diarrhea. Diagnostic procedures and tests include colonoscopy, barium enema study, and stool for occult blood, ova, parasites, toxins, bacteria.

Management is symptomatic and involves low residue/bland dietary inclusions if the source is infection or inflammation of the tract, or high fiber/bulk dietary inclusions to prevent diverticular disease and treat irritable bowel syndrome. Also, fluid intake of up to 2,500-3,000 mL./day is encouraged to replace losses. Antidiarrheal, antimicrobial, and antispasmodic drug therapy can also be administered.

Dietary Implications:

Clear liquid diet is given for 24-48 hours followed by a low residue/bland diet in acute diarrheal conditions

Provide or avoid fiber inclusion depending on cause and ability to tolerate

Avoid highly seasoned, fried, or raw foods, rich desserts, and alcohol

Add foods with high fluid content when possible

Add fiber-containing foods to casseroles, cooked vegetables, and soups if chewing and swallowing problems are present

Exchange Lists for Low Residue/Bland and High Fiber/Bulk Diets

Low Residue/Bland

Bread/Cereal:

White bread, rolls, crackers; rice, pasta products; cooked cereals, dry cereal without bran

Dairy Products:

Limited milk and milk products; cottage, American, cheddar cheeses; butter, margarine; eggs except fried

Meat:

Lean, tender, ground, broiled, baked, or stewed meats; poultry without skin; liver, crisp bacon; canned tuna or salmon

Vegetable:

Tender cooked vegetables; vegetable juices; vegetable broth, cream soups

Fruit:

Strained fruit juices; canned/stewed fruits without skins; applesauce, ripe banana

Miscellaneous:

All beverages except alcohol; oil, mayonnaise; custards, puddings; sherbet, plain ice cream; angel food, sponge cake, plain cookies; sugar, vinegar, lemon juice, spices if tolerated

High Fiber/Bulk

See Constipation for fiber/bulk inclusions for exchanges

Fluid/Electrolyte Imbalance

General Information:

Water is responsible for 50% of body weight in the older adult and must be replaced daily in the same amounts that are lost. Intake consists of water and other fluids, fluids contained in foods eaten, and water produced by oxidation. Water balance is regulated by water and sodium homeostasis and controlled by the kidneys. Because kidney function decreases with aging, older adults are more prone to fluid and electrolyte imbalances and dehydration. Sodium losses (hyponatremia) result from depletion of fluid volume caused by excesses in water loss and are usually associated with vomiting and diarrhea as well as drug therapy (diuretics). Sodium increases (hypernatremia) result from an inadequate intake of water and elevated temperature and are usually associated with vomiting and diarrhea as well as an impaired thirst mechanism. Underlying cardiac and renal failure disorders can also lead to sodium deficiency or excesses. Diagnostic tests include serum sodium and osmolality, BUN and Hct, and urinary specific gravity.

Management includes increased fluid intake and dietary sodium replacement (250 mg/serving) if levels are 126-135 mEq/L or IV replacement if levels <125 mEq/L.

Dietary Implications:

Normal sodium losses are about 115 mg/day and 500 mg/day satisfies daily need; intake should be limited to 2,400 mg/day

Sodium restriction can vary according to individual: mild (2,500-4,500 mg/day), moderate (1,000-2,000 mg/day)

Equivalency of sodium chloride (table salt) to sodium is 1 tsp or 5 g = 2,000 mg (40% of 5 g)

Salt is not added to foods or in food preparation and salt shaker is removed from the tray in sodium restricted diets

Sodium can be restricted (<50 mg/serving) in renal and cardiovascular diseases if excess fluid volume is a problem

Fluid intake can be increased to 2,000-2,500 mL/24 hour unless fluid restricted diet is prescribed; fluids can be limited to 800-1,000 mL/24 hour in chronic renal failure or chronic heart failure

Exchange Lists for Foods High or Low in Sodium

High Sodium

Bread/Cereal:

Commercial granola cereals; instant cooked, bran type cereals; saltine crackers, pretzels; pancake, waffle mixes, Bisquick; baking powder biscuits, muffins; cornbread, nutbread; rice or pasta mixes

Dairy Products:

Regular cheeses (natural, processed, cream)

Meat:

Smoked or cured meats (bacon, ham, sausage, hot dogs, cold cuts, salt pork); shellfish, sardines, herring, anchovies, caviar

Canned tuna, salmon, mackerel; bouillon cubes or dehydrated soups

Vegetable:

Cooked, frozen, canned vegetables; sauerkraut; canned vegetable juices; French fried potatoes, potato chips

Low Sodium

Unsalted breads, pasta; rice, puffed rice; shredded wheat

Salt free cheeses; low sodium whole or dry milk

Fresh meat, chicken, fish; low sodium frozen seafood

Fresh vegetables; low sodium frozen vegetables

Fruit:

Fresh, canned fruits   Fresh, canned fruits

Miscellaneous:

Salad dressings, mayonnaise, dips;   Unsalted popcorn; beverages; low
salted nuts or seeds; pizza, pot   sodium seasonings; salt substitute
pies; bottled, canned sodas, soft
drinks; olives, pickles, salted
popcorn; meat tenderizers, MSG,
soy sauce, mustard, chili and
steak sauces, horseradish,
barbecue sauce

Nausea

General Information:

Nausea is a condition or symptom resulting from injury or irritation to the gastric mucosa, or distention of the duodenum. Any underlying gastrointestinal condition that exerts tension on the stomach wall, lower esophagus, or duodenum can cause nausea. It can predispose to vomiting and a possible nutritional and fluid deficit. Decreased gastric motility resulting in stasis of contents, distasteful sights or odors, or drugs that stimulate the chemoreceptor trigger zone can cause vomiting. Diagnostic procedures and tests include gastroscopy.

Management of nausea and vomiting includes dietary restrictions, a clear liquid diet, increased fluid intake of up to 2,500 mL/day, and antiemetic, antacid, anticholinergic drug therapy.

Dietary Implications

Maintain NPO status until nausea (and vomiting) subside

Provide an environment of privacy and reduced stimuli

Encourage fluids, offer hard clear candies to relieve thirst

Avoid alcohol and other irritating liquids

Exchange Lists for Anti-Nausea Foods and Clear Liquid Diet

Clear Liquids

Fruit:

Clear fruit juices (apple, cranberry, grape), strained lemonade

Broth:

Bouillon, consommé

Desserts:

Plain gelatin, hard, clear candies, popsicles, fruit flavored ices

Beverage:

Ginger ale, water, tea, decaffeinated coffee, noncarbonated soda

Miscellaneous:

Honey, sugar, salt, Gatorade

Anti-Nausea Foods

White crackers; dry cereal without milk; plain mashed white potato; any dry food tolerated

Oral Mucositis/Stomatitis

General Information:

Oral mucositis or stomatitis is a condition or symptom resulting from the effects of medications (chemotherapeutic agents) on the oral mucous membrane. It affects oral intake of foods and fluids and is managed by emphasis on a high protein/caloric and soft diet with supplemental offerings. Fluids are encouraged to treat the dry mouth and viscous saliva associated with this condition.

Dietary Implications:

Dietary modifications include avoidance of spicy foods, very hot or cold foods, citrus foods and fluids, or alcohol

Soft, bland foods can be offered to prevent additional irritation of mucosa and pain

Exchange Lists for Mechanical Soft Foods and Low Residue/Bland Diet

Mechanical Soft

Bread/Cereal:

Plain white, whole wheat, rye bread without seeds; all pastas, rice; cooked cereals; plain cakes, cookies

Dairy Products:

Milk and milk products; cream, cottage, mild cheddar cheeses; egg, butter, eggnog, yogurt

Meat:

Chopped, ground, pureed, or tender meats and poultry; baked fish

Vegetable:

Cooked or canned tender vegetables; all vegetable juices; vegetable soups (plain and cream); potatoes, hominy

Fruit:

Fruit slushes; cooked or canned fruits without skins; ripe banana

Dessert:

Puddings, custards, gelatin; smooth ice cream, sherbet

Miscellaneous:

Sugar, honey, syrup, clear jelly; vegetable oils, salad dressings; white sauce; broth, consommé

Low Residue/Bland

See Diarrhea for low residue/bland inclusions for exchanges

Wound Healing

General Information:

Wound healing is the process of tissue repair that involves a course of initial inflammatory response, tissue regeneration, and finally scar formation. In the older adult, wounds result from surgical incision, trauma, or decubitus ulcer. The major nutritional considerations important to wound healing include water, protein (increase to 1.5 g/kg/day), vitamin A (increase to 25,000 IU/day), vitamins C, B_6 (increase in proportion to protein intake), and calories (increase to 3,500/day with 50% or more carbohydrate).

Management involves the sterile procedures performed to care for the wound and the provision of the additional nutrients administered in the diet or as oral supplements. Complications include wound infection, wound disruption, or skin irritation and breakdown. Diagnostic test considerations include wound culture to identify infectious agents.

Dietary Implications

Additional vitamins and minerals can be included such as iron, folic acid, and zinc; deficiencies of these substances are sometimes responsible for slowing wound healing by causing impaired protein and collagen synthesis, and decreased oxygen transport to the wound site

Decreased circulation common in the older adult can slow the healing process, as an adequate blood supply is necessary to transport nutrients to the wound

Malnutrition will impact healing: protein deficiency affects collagen and leukocyte synthesis; fat and carbohydrate deficiency causes the breakdown of protein needed for tissue building and energy

Those at risk for decubitus ulcer should have nutritional support and supplementation if dietary intake is inadequate

Exchange Lists for Foods High in Protein, Calories, Vitamin C

Protein	Calories	Vitamin C
Bread/Cereal:		
	All breads, rolls, pasta, cereals, pastries, cakes, pancakes, waffles, cookies	
Dairy Products:		
Milk and milk products, cottage and other cheeses, egg, yogurt	Whole milk and milk products, sour cream, all cheeses, egg, butter, ice cream	
Meat:		
All poultry, beef, veal, pork, lamb, fish	All poultry, meats, fish	
Vegetable:		
Lentils, soybeans, dried beans	Potatoes, yams, corn, dried beans	Tomatoes and tomato juice, white potatoes, dark green leafy vegetables, raw green/red peppers, cole slaw
Fruit:		
All fresh fruits	All fresh, canned fruit	Orange, grapefruit, cranberry fruits and juices, strawberries, muskmelon

Nuts:

Peanut butter, peanuts, sunflower seeds, sesame seeds	Peanut butter

Miscellaneous:

Mayonnaise, salad dressings, sauces, gravies	Mayonnaise, salad dressings, sauces, gravies, honey

CHAPTER VIII

PROCEDURES TO PROVIDE NUTRITION

A.   Oral Feedings
           Feeding/Assisting with Meals
           Use of Assistive Aids

B.   Enteral Tube Feedings
           Nasogastric Tube Feeding
           Tips for Nasogastric Tube Care
           Tips for Nasogastric Tube Feeding
           Gastrostomy Tube Feeding
           Tips for Gastrostomy Tube Care
           Tips for Gastrostomy Tube Feeding
           Types of Formulae
           Common Commercial Formulae
           Formula Preparation

C.   Total Parenteral Nutrition
           Tips for Total Parenteral Nutrition
           Administration, Care, and
           Maintenance

D.   Intravenous Fluid/Nutritional Therapy
           (Peripheral)
           Tips for Intravenous Fluid/Nutrition
           Administration, Care, and
           Maintenance

Oral Feedings

Adequate nutritional intake by the older adult is influenced by physiologic and psychosocial problems.

Physiologic problems include:

1. Dental disorders, e.g., tooth loss, tooth pain, periodontal disease, poor fitting dentures.

2. Oral disorders, e.g., stomatitis, dry mouth, chewing problems, loss of tongue strength, deteriorating oral structures, change in gustatory and olfactory perception.

3. Esophageal disorders, e.g., dysphagia, pain, pyrosis, gastroesophageal reflux, hiatal hernia, tumor.

4. Gastric disorders, e.g., nausea, vomiting, anorexia, pain, belching, dyspepsia, inflammation, peptic ulcer, tumor.

5. Intestinal disorders, e.g., diarrhea, constipation, pain, malabsorption, tumor, inflammation, diverticular disease, obstruction.

6. Liver, pancreas, and biliary tract disorders, e.g., inflammation, liver cirrhosis, tumor, diabetes mellitus, chronic gallbladder disease.

7. Other impairments, e.g., visual, paralysis, facial muscles, hand-arm coordination, inability to use and manipulate eating utensils, fatigue, effect of medications on appetite and nutrition.

Psychosocial problems include:

1. Dementia, e.g., confusion, disorientation, memory deficit, distractibility, impaired judgement.

2. Attitude, e.g., isolation, loneliness, loss of interest, apathy, refusal to eat.

3. Grieving, depression, insomnia.

4. Ignorance/noncompliance with cultural and/or special dietary requirements.

Feeding/Assisting with Meals:

Older adults sometimes are unable to assume complete independence in the self-feeding activity. This can be a temporary disability, as in situations where strength and physical capabilities are completely or partially restored by rehabilitation therapy. It can, however, be permanent as in organic brain disease, stroke, or neuromuscular diseases.

Feeding can develop into a problem for both resident and staff member responsible for feeding or assisting with meals. (See Age-Related Tips to Promote Nutrition.)

Steps to follow for a successful feeding experience include:

1.   Offer and assist to use bathroom, commode, bedpan prior to meals.

2.   Assist with washing of hands prior to meals, mouth care if needed.

3.   Position upright in bed or chair, preferably in a communal setting or, if alone, with a radio or TV on; if feeding in bed, support the head to prevent hyperextension.

4.   Provide a comfortable, orderly, odor free environment; prevent any interruptions at mealtime.

5.   Ensure that correct and culturally appropriate diet is offered.

6.   Check dietary inclusions for foods that are palatable and of proper consistency if swallowing is a problem; finger foods can be eaten using less energy.

7.   Place tray in front of and within reach at an appropriate height, check temperature of the foods.

8.   Display patience, smile, and avoid a rushing attitude; praise all efforts and encourage continued independent feeding.

9.   To provide assistance, prepare tray by cutting meat in medium sized bites, open cartons and packages, pour liquids and sprinkle condiments, spread butter/margarine on bread, position and secure napkin on chest.

10. Provide assistive utensils for self-feeding in those with some functional loss.

11. To provide complete feeding, prepare tray as above, offer small to medium sized bites of each food and allow time to chew and swallow, offer fluids if desired; allow opportunity for selection of food and amounts.

12. Always explain what foods are presented and cater to individual preferences and culturally symbolic foods when possible.

13. Talk and socialize while feeding.

14. If refused to be fed, allow to feed self no matter how awkward; protect clothing from spills.

15. Emphasize inclusions of foods high in protein, energy, vitamin/mineral content since fatigue can terminate a meal with limited amounts ingested.

16. Consider liberalizing meal plan when intake is poor.

Use of Assistive Aids:

1. Assess physical limitations and their causes.

2. Assess use of dominant hand, arm, or opposite hand and arm, hand-mouth coordination.

3. Provide assistive aids as appropriate:

   Suction dishes, bowls, cups to prevent movement on tray.

   Dish with broad edge to push food against when using a utensil.

   Lightweight cups with a small opening for drinking and large handle for grasping and holding.

   Extra-thick handles on utensils for easier grasp, can be built up with foam and tape.

   Extension handles and adjustable shafts on forks, spoons, knives; swivel spoon or fork, rocker knife.

   Cuff-mounted utensils that slip over the hand eliminating the need to grasp utensils.

Glass holder, adhesive tape on glass to prevent slipping.

Tilting glass holder and straw to allow for holding straw while glass is stationary.

Sandwich holder to assist in bringing sandwich to mouth.

Non-slip placemats, napkin large enough to tuck in at neckline and protect clothing.

Lap board if in a wheelchair.

Federal/Community Nutrition Programs:

1.   Meals on Wheels

2.   Food Stamps

3.   Salvation Army

4.   Church groups and clubs

5.   Others related to the aging population

Enteral Tube Feedings

Nasogastric Tube Feeding:

Tube feedings are administered via gravity into the stomach or small intestine through a tube inserted into the nose (nasogastric) or mouth (orogastric). This method is usually used for feedings when a resident is unable to ingest food orally but still maintains bowel function. Feedings consist of a liquid formula that is nutritionally adequate (proteins, carbohydrates, fats) and prepared commercially. Amounts and frequency depend on individual nutritional and fluid needs and health status. Continuous feedings can be administered by gravity or infusion pump. Type and size of tube inserted depends on placement in the stomach or intestine and whether the feedings are administered by gravity or infusion pump. The most likely candidates for this procedure are those with dental and oral structure deterioration problems, gastrointestinal disease, mental confusion, neurologic deficits, paralysis, anorexia, depression, extreme weakness, or comatose state. It requires normal gastric motility and gastric outlet function.

Tips for Nasogastric Tube Care:

1. Assess for type and size of tube to be inserted and route, nares for deviation and patency, presence of gag reflex.

2. Assess for nutritional status, long- or short-term use, continuous or intermittent feedings.

3. Place in sitting or high-Fowler's, position with pillow behind shoulders.

4. Place towel over the chest and provide a glass of water and straw to hold.

5. Use disposable gloves and clean technique to perform care procedures.

6. Measure the length of tube (earlobe to xyphoid process) to be inserted and mark with tape, lubricate with water or water soluble lubricant prior to insertion.

7. Ensure pliability of a plastic tube by warming in warm water.

8. Coil tube around hand and gently and steadily insert tip of tube into nares in a downward and lateral movement.

9. Terminate insertion of the tube if met with resistance, remove and reinsert in the opposite nares.

10. Rotate tube during insertion and when pharynx is reached, request swallowing a small amount of water while continuing to insert the tube; insert with each swallow until marked length is reached.

11. If gagging continues, check pharynx with a flashlight and tongue blade—tubing can be coiled in back of the mouth or trachea.

12. Check placement by aspirating contents with a syringe, injecting air and listening for lung sounds indicating that tube is in the lungs.

13. Secure tube in place with the least amount of pressure to the nasal mucosa.

14. Clamp tubing and secure to clothing.

15. For long-term nasogastric feedings, rotate nares to prevent damage to mucosa from prolonged pressure and irritation; change tubing every 4 weeks.

16. Provide thorough mouth care 3-4 times/day; assess for dryness and discomfort.

17. Apply protective ointment to nares and lips to decrease irritation and dryness; clean any dry crusting from the tube; change tape daily or if wet or loose.

18. Use throat sprays or lozenges to relieve throat discomfort; give frequent sips of water, chewing gum or hard candy if permitted for dryness.

19. Include aspirate, irrigation fluid, and feedings in I&O measurement monitoring.

20. Administer at least 2,000 mL/day fluid intake and 1,600-1,800 mL caloric intake.

Tips for Nasogastric Tube Feeding:

1. Assess for type of formula, feeding times, amount and frequency, method of administration (gravity or pump).

2. Place in semi-Fowler's position and place towel over chest to protect clothing.

3. Unplug or unclamp tube and check placement by aspiration or injecting air and listening for sounds in stomach or lungs.

4. Aspirate for residual contents in stomach with a 60 mL syringe and, if less than 50% of last feeding, reinject aspirate and continue with gavage.

5. Attach syringe barrel to feeding tube and irrigate with 30 mL water to check for tube patency.

6. Pour formula into the barrel from the measured container and raise 12 inches above stomach level.

7.   Allow to flow by gravity and add more formula before barrel empties until all the measured amount has been given, adjust rate by raising or lowering the barrel containing the formula. Infuse each feeding over a 20-40 minute period.

8.   Flush the tube with 30-60 mL tap water to clear formula.

9.   Clamp or plug the tube end and maintain elevated position for 45 minutes.

10.   If feeding is continuous, pour prepared formula into a container and close top, attach administration set to container, remove air, attach to feeding tube, regulate drop rate with or without use of infusion pump, and check for residual and flush tube with 30 mL tap water every 8-12 hours.

11.   Assess for complications that can include: bacterial contamination caused by improper handling or storage of formula, distention and bloating caused by feeding at a rapid rate, nausea caused by delayed gastric emptying as motility is decreased and too much formula is given, aspiration caused by improper placement of tube, increased emptying of stomach and diarrhea caused by feeding that is too cold, diarrhea and dehydration caused by high osmolarity of feeding, high lactose concentration if intolerance is present, allergic reaction to formula.

Gastrostomy Tube Feeding:

Gastrostomy tube feeding is another method of administering feedings into the stomach by gravity. The gastrostomy is a surgically created abdominal opening into the stomach performed and used for long-term intermittent or continuous feedings. The stoma can contain a button with a mushroom type dome to secure the device under the skin and a plug that can be opened or closed at the surface of the skin. This button implantation is not likely to become displaced or develop leakage of the gastric contents as it contains an antireflux valve. It can also contain an inflatable tube inserted into the stomach and skin disk to secure the position of the tube. Formula used in the feedings are the same as for nasogastric tube feedings with amounts and frequency dependent on individual nutritional and fluid needs and health status. Those most likely to receive this method are the same as for nasogastric tube feedings.

Tips for Gastrostomy Tube Care:

1. Assess for type of device, amount and frequency of feedings, and nutritional status.

2. Use disposable gloves to perform care and procedures.

3. Perform insertion of gastrostomy button using a lubricated obturator; insert through the stoma; remove the obturator after the valve closes, check that the valve is closed, and close the plug at the skin surface until feeding time.

4. Perform insertion of balloon type gastrostomy tube by positioning the skin disk in position on the abdomen, insert the tube into the stoma up to the disk, inflating the balloon, and gently tugging on the tube to ensure anchoring.

5. Perform site care by removing dressing, cleansing the skin around the tube with antiseptic swabs followed by saline swabs, redressing with sterile gauze, securing tube for exposure when needed for feedings, taping dressing and tube in place.

6. Include feedings in I&O measurement monitoring.

Tips for Gastrostomy Tube Feeding:

1. Assess for type of formula, amount and frequency, method of administration (gravity or pump).

2. Place in semi-Fowler's position with drape site for privacy concerns.

3. Open the flexible plug and connect the tubing from the container of formula to the adaptor on the button, position the formula container 12 inches above the stoma site.

4. Unclamp the tubing and allow 20-40 minutes for the formula to flow into the stomach by gravity, adjust the rate by raising or lowering the formula container.

5. Add 30-60 mL of tap water before the container empties to clear the tubing and ensure that all the formula enters the stomach.

6. Disconnect the tubing from the adaptor and close the flexible plug.

7. If a balloon type of tube is in place, attach the syringe or tubing from a container of formula to the tube, allow to flow by gravity, follow by 30 mL of tap water before the container is empty to clear the tubing, and complete the procedure by removing the syringe or container.

8. Administer smaller amounts more frequently if resident complains of fullness.

9. Maintain the position for 45 minutes following the feeding.

10. Assess for the same complications outlined in nasogastric tube feeding.

Types of Formulae:

Commercially prepared formulated feeding are also known as formula diets for medical use, dietary supplements, and enteral feedings. They are available in cans in liquid form or packages in powder form, and are formulated to be nutrition-ally complete. They are also available for specific medical conditions such as renal failure, chronic obstructive pulmonary disease, liver dysfunction, and low sodium, or to supply additional calories, or a minimum of digestion.

Common Commercial Formulae

Name	Uses	Preparation	Total Calories/L
Ensure	Oral or Tube	Canned and powdered	1,060/Lactose free
Osmolite	Oral or Tube	Canned/No preparation	1,060/Lactose free; low osmolality
Sustacal	Oral or Tube	Canned and powdered	1,000
Vital	Oral or Tube	Powdered	1,000/Lactose free; low residue
Resource	Oral or Tube	Powdered	1,000/Lactose free/low residue

High Protein Modules: Casec
Promod

High Carbohydrate Modules: Polycose
Sumacal

High Fat Modules: Microlipid
MCT Oil

Low Protein: Nephro
Amin-Aid

Formula Preparation:

Liquid:

1.   Check container for cracks, leaks, and expiration date.

2.   Warm to room temperature by removing from the refrigerator 15 minutes prior to administration.

3.   Rinse top of can or bottle and dry with paper towel.

4.   Open container and pour proper amount into feeding container or a graduated container if measurement is necessary.

5.   Close or cover feeding container, refrigerate amount not used and record date and time opened. Discard unused portion within 24 hours.

6.   If administering via a syringe barrel by gravity, take the container with the measured amount to the bedside.

Powdered:

1.   Gradually add appropriate amount of powder to appropriate amount of liquid and mix with a blender or mixer to dissolve.

2.   Prepare only the amount needed for 24 hours, label with the date and time, and refrigerate the unused portion.

3.   Pour proper amount into feeding container or graduated container if using a syringe barrel to administer by gravity.

4.   Warm to room temperature following removal from refrigerator, as previously outlined, prior to administration.

5.   Take the container with the measured amount of formula to the bedside.

Total Parenteral Nutrition

Total parenteral nutrition (TPN) is the intravenous infusion of specially prepared solutions to provide essential nutrients for long periods of time when oral, tube, or subcutaneous intravenous therapy is inadequate or contraindicated. It is administered via a central vein (usually the subclavian) using an indwelling catheter inserted and anchored by the physician with placement in the superior vena cava or right atrium. It can also be administered through a right atrial catheter (RAC) inserted through an incision in the right upper chest. All nutritional requirements including amino acids, glucose, fats, vitamins, minerals, electrolytes, and trace elements can be supplied with this method. Intralipid solution can be included in TPN if therapy is to be given longer than 2 weeks and requirement cannot be met by feedings but should be used with caution in those with pancreas, liver, or pulmonary disorders. Candidates for this type of therapy include those with malnutrition or cachexia caused by chronic diseases, debilitating diseases such as cancer, renal or hepatic failure, and gastrointestinal disorders that affect ingestion, digestion, or absorption of nutrients.

A possible example of the composition of 1 L of TPN solution includes:

42.5 g	Amino Acids
50 mEq	Sodium
10 mEq	Calcium
10 mM	Phosphate
35 mEq	Potassium
8 mEq	Magnesium
0.1 mg	Manganese
1.0 mg	Zinc
0.4 mg	Copper
4% g	Chromium

0.5 mg	Folic Acid
550 mg	Ascorbic Acid
	B Complex Vitamins
3.5 mL	Multivitamin Preparation Added/Week

Calories calculated to specific needs

Intralipid solution includes:

2.5 g/kg/day is the usual amount administered with the solution composed of soybean oil, egg yolk phosphatide and glycerol.

Tips for TPN Administration, Care, and Maintenance:

1. Assess type and amount of solutions, rate of administration, catheter insertion site, and type of catheter.

2. Assess general nutritional and health status and reason for TPN.

3. Utilize sterile technique when performing all procedures associated with TPN administration, universal precautions when disposing of all used supplies.

4. Check prepared solutions, ensuring that solutions in bags are clear and free of precipitate or discoloration. Confirm agreement with orders and check date.

5. Prepare tubing set-up, connect to solution, and administer TPN safely and at correct volume and time via an infusion pump set at a rate in mL/hour.

6. Prepare tubing set-up for fat emulsion if to be given, connect to infusion below the filter via a Y injection site on the TPN tubing, and administer following TPN solution via the pump set at the correct rate and time in ml/hour.

7. Change dressings, solutions, and tubing according to agency policy.

8. If RAC is in place, remove dressing and tape, prepare cap connector with Betadine and alcohol, irrigate catheter as needed, use special clamp on catheter if needed, connect tubing set-up to catheter and tape to prevent leakage, set pump at correct rate and time in mL/hour, provide any special site care; discontinue, replace cap, irrigate catheter, and redress as needed.

9. Monitor drop rate, catheter and tubing patency, vital signs, I&O during the infusion, weight daily for fluid and caloric changes.

10. Monitor urinary glucose and ketones q4h, serum potassium, sodium, calcium, protein, lipid levels, and nitrogen balance according to agency policy to note possible complications.

11. Assess insertion site for redness, swelling, pain, drainage indicating infection.

12. Notify physician if catheter becomes dislodged or displaced.

13. Assess for complications including hyperglycemia caused by excessive rate of infusion, excessive total load of infusion, inadequate or persistent insulin response; metabolic acidosis caused by excessive chloride and monohydrochloride content of amino acid solution; azotemia caused by excessive amino acid infusion; thrombocytopenia and poor wound healing caused by inadequate essential fatty acids; hypocalcemia and hypophosphatemia caused by inadequate amounts of calcium and phosphorus in TPN solution; hypo or hypervitaminosis caused by excessive or deficiency of vitamins.

14. Evaluate for under or overfeeding (weight and nutritional status parameter changes).

Intravenous Fluid/Nutritional Therapy (Peripheral)

Intravenous (IV) fluid/nutritional therapy is given to replace and maintain fluid and nutritional needs by peripheral infusion. It is usually reserved for short-term nutritional support by administration of fluid, calories (glucose) and mineral salts (sodium chloride, potassium, magnesium, calcium, and phosphate) according to specific needs. One L of 5% dextrose in water (D5W) equals 170 kcal and one L of 10% dextrose (D5NS). Common indications for therapy include prevention of dehydration caused by vomiting, diarrhea, excessive fluid losses from other routes, increased fluid requirements from fever or increased metabolism, inability to ingest fluids orally, and need for electrolyte replacement and restoration of plasma volume.

Solution	Contents	Uses
D5W (5% dextrose in water)	5 g dextrose/100 mL	Provides fluids/ short-term nutrition, prevents dehydration
D₅ 1/2 NS (5% dextrose in 0.45% normal saline)	5 g dextrose/100 mL	Replaces fluid and sodium losses, promotes diuresis
NS (0.9% sodium chloride)	14 mEq/L sodium; 154 mEq/L chloride	Fluid losses
Ringers solution	14 mEq/L sodium; 155 mEq/L chloride; 4 mEq/L potassium; 4 mEq/L calcium	Replaces fluid and electrolytes in vomiting, diarrhea, dehydration
Lactated Ringers	130 mEq/L sodium; 109 mEq/L chloride; 4 mEq/l potassium; 4 mEq/L calcium	Dehydration, restoration of fluid balance

Calculation of drip rate:

The rate is calculated using the amount of fluid to be infused, amount of time to infuse the fluid, number of drops/mL delivered by the infusion set (drop factor). Sets can be calibrated in 10 or 15 drops/mL (macrodrip) or 60 drops/mi (microdrip).

Example using the formula method of calculation:

Order:
1 L D_5W to be infused over 24 hours
(drop factor of set is 15 drops/mL)

Conversion:
1 L = 1,000 mL, and 1 hour = 60 min;
24 hour = 60 x 24 = 1,440 min

Formula Method:

$$\frac{1{,}000mL \times 15\ drops}{1{,}440\ min} = \frac{1{,}500\ drops}{144\ min} = 10.4\ or\ 10\ ^{drops}/_{min}$$

Ratio-Proportion Method:
1,000 mL: 1,440 min :: x mL: 1 min

$$\frac{\cancel{1{,}440min}\ X}{\cancel{1{,}440min}} = \frac{1{,}000mL}{1{,}440min}$$

$$X = 0.61\ ^{mL}/_{min}$$

$$0.61\ ^{mL}/_{min} \times 15\ ^{drops}/_{mL} = 9.15\ or\ 9\ ^{drops}/_{min}$$

Dimensional Analysis Method:

$$\frac{1{,}000\ \cancel{mL}}{24\ \cancel{hr}} \times \frac{15\ drops}{1\ \cancel{mL}} \times \frac{1\ \cancel{hr}}{60\ min} = \frac{250\ drops}{24\ min} = 10.4\ or\ 10\ ^{drops}/_{min}$$

Tips for Intravenous Fluid/Nutrition Administration, Care, and Maintenance:

1. Assess type and amount of solution, rate of administration, type of set-up and cannula or device.

2. Assess reason for IV therapy, fluid and nutritional needs.

3. Utilize sterile technique when performing all procedures associated with IV therapy; universal precautions when disposing of used supplies.

4. Check solution for clarity and absence of precipitate or discoloration, container for damage, expiration date.

5. Prepare solutions and set-up, label container with date, calculate drip rate correctly in drops/min or mL/hour.

6. Administer fluids and manually adjust drop and volume rate or use control device, monitor rate q1h to maintain rate and volume.

7. Monitor infusion site for infiltration (pain, swelling, leakage around insertion site, lack of flow), cannula displacement, tubing for kinking and patency, need for dressing change.

8. Immobilize limb with armboard and remove to exercise q2-4h.

9. Monitor for I&O q4-8h and electrolyte imbalance as appropriate.

10. Change solution, tubing set-up, site as needed or according to agency policy.

Chapter IX

DRUGS RELATED TO THE GASTROINTESTINAL SYSTEM
AND NUTRITION/DIET THERAPY

A. Analgesics
B. Antacids
C. Antianemics
D. Antidiabetics
E. Antidiarrheals
F. Antiemetics
G. Antiflatulants
H. Antilipemics
I. Antimicrobials
J. Bronchodilators
K. Cardiovascular Agents
L. Digestants
M. Diuretics
N. Electrolytes
O. Histamine H$_2$ Blockers
P. Laxatives
Q. Psychotherapeutic Agents
R. Vitamins/Minerals

Older adults have more chronic diseases and health problems and take more prescribed and over-the-counter (OTC) drugs than any other age group. It is not uncommon for these individuals to have more than one disorder and have several drugs prescribed. They are more likely to experience adverse reactions because of the number of drugs taken and the decreased function of organs involved in absorption, distribution, metabolism, and elimination brought about by the aging process. Medication regimens can affect nutritional status by interfering with ingestion, digestion, and absorption of nutrients. Also, foods can affect the drug action by interfering with metabolism and absorption or containing substances that have pharmacologic action that interact with drugs taken.

Analgesics

Indications:	Mild to severe headache, oral pain, arthritic pain, other situations; aspirin to reduce risk of heart attack or cerebral accident
Narcotic:	Codeine (Methylmorphine) - moderate pain relief; oxycodone (Percodan) - moderate to severe pain relief
GI tract side effects:	Nausea, vomiting, constipation
Nutritional side effects:	None
Interactions with other drugs:	Increases CNS depression by alcohol, sedatives, antihistamines, and antidepressants; decreases analgesic effect by pentazocine and nalbuphine; withdrawal can be initiated by nalbuphine, buprenorphine, pentazocine

Non-narcotic:	Aspirin (ASA) - mild pain relief, antipyretic, anti-inflammatory; acetaminophen (Tylenol)- mild pain relief, antipyretic; ibuprofen (Motrin)- mild to moderate pain relief, antipyretic, anti-inflammatory
GI tract side effects:	Anorexia, nausea, vomiting, dyspepsia, constipation, gastro-intestinal distress and/or bleeding, dry mouth; gastritis and bleeding leading to anemic disorder with aspirin therapy
Nutritional side effects:	Aspirin - decreases folate and vitamin C levels with chronic use; acetaminophen - high intake of carbohydrates can decrease absorption; increases loss of ascorbic acid in urine
Interactions with other drugs:	Anti-inflammatory agents - enhances action of anticoagulants, oral antidiabetics, phenytoin, probenecid, tetracyclines, phenyl-butazone; increases nephro and hepatotoxicity when taken with other drugs that are toxic to these organs

Antacids

Indications:	Gastritis, indigestion, heartburn, hiatal hernia/esophageal reflux; short-term treatment for constipation with magnesium hydroxide
Aluminum/magnesium hydroxide (Maalox, Mylanta):	Combined to reduce gastrointestinal side effects; neutralizes action of gastric acid by raising pH of secretions, inactivates pepsin; can contain an antiflatulant

Nutritional side effects:	Sodium and sugar content should be determined for those on sodium and carbohydrate restricted diets, as some antacids contain varying amounts of these substances
	Calcium content should be determined as milk-alkali syndrome can develop with milk inclusion in the diet and long-term therapy
Interactions with other drugs:	Decreases absorption of iron, isoniazid, tetracyclines, phenothiazines; doses that alkalinize the urine can decrease quinidine, amphetamine, and salicylate excretion leading to toxicity
Aluminum hydroxide (Amphojel):	Neutralizes gastric acid, inactivates pepsin, binds with phosphate in the tract
GI tract side effects:	Constipation, possible bowel obstruction
Nutritional side effects:	Phosphorus deficiency can develop with long-term diet low in protein and phosphorus; vitamin A and B_1 deficiency can develop with impaired absorption (see Aluminum/Magnesium Hydroxide)
Interactions with other drugs:	Decreases absorption of iron, isoniazid, fluoroquinolones, tetracyclines, chlorpromazines; blood levels of salicylates can decrease, and levels of quinidine and amphetamines can increase with increase in urinary pH
Magnesium hydroxide (Milk of Magnesia):	Neutralizes gastric acid, acts as a laxative by drawing water into the colon

GI side effects:	Diarrhea, nausea, abdominal cramping, dehydration
Nutritional side effects:	Reduces iron and phosphate absorption (see Aluminum/ Magnesium Hydroxide)
Interactions with other drugs:	Enhances action of neuromuscular blocking agents and decreases absorption of fluoroquinolones; toxicity possible in those with renal impairment
Magaldrate (Riopan):	Combined aluminum and magnesium preparation; neutralizes gastric acid and inactivates pepsin
Nutritional side effects:	(See Aluminum/Magnesium Hydroxide)
Interactions with other drugs:	Same interactions listed in aluminum hydroxide

Antianemics

Indications:	Prevent or treat iron or folic acid deficiency anemia, pernicious anemia
Iron preparations (Iron dextran, ferrous fumarate, ferrous gluconate, ferrous sulfate):	Replenish iron stores needed for hemoglobin production
GI tract side effects:	(Iron dextran) Nausea, vomiting
	(Ferrous preparations) Nausea, epigastric pain, diarrhea, constipation, dark color of stools, upper gastrointestinal bleeding
Nutritional side effects:	Coordinate dietary intake with oral supplemental iron administration; decrease of iron absorption of up to 1/2 with food intake

Interactions with other drugs:	Decreases absorption of iron by antacids and tetracycline and increases absorption by vitamin C; decreases absorption of tetracycline, penicillamine or fluoroquinolones with iron administration
	(Iron dextran) Desired response by parenteral administration can be impaired by vitamin E and chloramphenicol
Cyanocobalamin (Vitamin B$_{12}$):	Supply this vitamin needed for red blood cell production
Interactions with other drugs:	Depletes B$_{12}$ by cimeditine that decreases gastric secretions
Folic Acid (Vitamin B$_9$):	Supply or replenish this vitamin needed for red blood cell production
Interactions with drugs:	Decreases absorption of folic acid by sulfasalazine; inhibits action by sulfonamides, methotrexate; increases need for folic acid with administration of phenytoin, estrogens, glucocorticoids

Antidiabetics

Indications:	Treat diabetes mellitus
Sulfonylureas (Glipizide, Tolbutaimide):	Control blood sugar in type 2 diabetes when diet therapy alone is insufficient
GI side effects:	Nausea, vomiting, abdominal cramping, diarrhea, hepatitis
Nutritional side effects:	Coordinate with dietary intake to prevent hypo or hyperglycemic reactions; weight gain

Interactions with other drugs:	Alcohol can shorten the time of the drug's action and cause hyperglycemia; reduce drug effectiveness by thiazides, glucocorticoids, rifampin; enhances drug effectiveness by androgens, clofibrate, monoamine oxidase inhibitors, sulfonamides, anticoagulants, phenylbutazone, salicylates; absent hypoglycemic symptoms with administration of adrenergic blocking agents
Acarbose (Precose):	As adjunct to diet for control of blood sugar in type 2 diabetes when diet alone insufficient; may also be used in combination with a sulfonylurea
GI side effects:	Retards the breakdown of carbohydrates and can cause flatulence, abdominal pain, diarrhea
Nutritional side effects:	Used alone should not cause hypoglycemia or hyperinsulinemia which can contribute to weight gain
	Used with sulfonylureas may have increased hypoglycemic response
	Hypoglycemia will not respond to orange juice or pop; glucose or dextrose tablets are effective
Interactions with other drugs:	The following drugs tend to produce hyperglycemia and may lead to loss of blood sugar control: thiazides and diuretics; corticosteroids; thyroid drugs; estrogens; phenytoin; nicotinic acid; calcium channel blockers

Metformin (glucophage):	Controls blood sugar in type 2 diabetes either alone or in conjunction with a sulfonylurea
GI side effects:	Diarrhea; nausea; abdominal bloating; flatulence; anorexia
Nutritional side effects:	May cause interference in B_{12} absorption
	Does not cause hypoglycemia when used alone under usual circumstances
Interactions with other drugs:	Increases blood levels with furosemide, nifedipine, cemetidine
	Alcohol potentiates effect of metformin on lactate metabolism
	Thiazides, diuretics, corticosteroids, thyroid drugs, estrogens, phenytoin, nicotinic acid, and calcium channel blockers can produce hyperglycemia and lead to loss of blood sugar control
Troglitazon (Rezulin):	Type 2 diabetes when greater than 30 units of insulin per day as multiple injections fail to adequately control hyperglycemia
	May be used as initial therapy
	Most effective in combination with sulfonylureas
GI side effects:	None
Nutritional side effects:	May require reduction in insulin dose to prevent hypoglycemia
Interactions with other drugs:	Reduces effectiveness of oral contraceptives; decreases efficacy of terfanadine
	Cholestyramine reduces absorption and thus efficacy

Insulin **_(rapid, intermediate,_** **_long acting):_**	Pancreatic hormone to control blood sugar in diabetes type 1, and in type 2 if diet and oral hypoglycemic therapy has failed
Nutritional side effects:	Coordinate with dietary intake and timing with type and timing of insulin
	Infection or extreme stress can cause need to change dietary and medication regimens
Interactions with other drugs:	Increases insulin requirements by thiazide diuretics, thyroid drugs, estrogens, rifampin, alcohol, glucocorticoids; decreases insulin requirements by salicylates, anticoagulants, anabolic steroids, tricyclic antidepressants, phenylbutazone

Antidiarrheals

Indications:	Treat acute or chronic mild to moderate diarrhea
Diphenoxylate/atropine **_(Lomotil):_**	Reduces intestinal motility and relief of diarrhea
GI side effects:	Constipation, possible fecal impaction, dry mouth, paralytic ileus
Nutritional side effects:	Reduces absorption of nutrients in intestines with prolonged use; fluid and electrolyte imbalance
Interactions with other drugs:	Enhances CNS depression by alcohol, narcotic analgesics, sedatives, hypnotics; enhances anticholinergic effect by tricyclic antidepressants, disopyramide, hypertensive crisis with MAO inhibitors

Loperamide (Immodium):   Reduces intestinal motility and relief of diarrhea

GI side effects: Nausea, constipation, dry mouth

Nutritional side effects: Reduces absorption of nutrients in intestines with prolonged use; fluid and electrolyte imbalance

Interactions with other drugs: Enhances CNS depression by alcohol, narcotics, sedatives, hypnotics, antihistamines; enhances anticholinergic effect by tricyclic antidepressants and antihistamines

Kaolin/pectin (Kaopectate):   Reduces fluids in feces and relief of diarrhea

GI side effects: Constipation

Nutritional side effects: Reduces absorption of nutrients in intestines with prolonged use; fluid and electrolyte imbalance

Interactions with other drugs: Decreases absorption of chloroquine, digoxin

Antiemetics

Indications: Prevent or treat nausea and vomiting by depressing the chemoreceptor trigger zone of the CNS

Promethazine (Phenergan):   Prevents nausea and vomiting

GI side effects: Constipation, dry mouth, hepatitis, anorexia

Nutritional side effects: Continuous or intermittent nausea and/or vomiting of dietary intake can result in altered ingestion, digestion; nutritional deficits/fluid and electrolyte imbalance, especially in a debilitated older adult

Interactions with other drugs:	Enhances CNS depression by alcohol, narcotics, sedatives, hypnotics, antianxiety agents; enhance anticholinergic effect with antihistamines, atropine, haloperidol, antidepressants, phenothiazines, quinidine

Prochlorperazine (Compazine):

	Controls nausea and vomiting
GI side effects:	Anorexia, dry mouth, constipation, paralytic ileus, hepatitis
Nutritional side effects:	(See promethazine)
Interactions with other drugs:	Enhances CNS depression and anticholinergic effect by drugs listed for promethazine; decreases absorption by and interferes with symptoms of toxicity of lithium; decreases absorption by antacids; reduces benefits of levadopa; causes hypotension by administration of antihypertensives or nitrates

Metoclopramide (Reglan):

	Decreases symptoms associated with gastric stasis, controls nausea and vomiting
GI side effects:	Nausea, dry mouth, constipation, diarrhea
Nutritional side effects:	(See promethazine)
Interactions with other drugs:	Enhances CNS depression by drugs listed for above drugs; decreases absorption of any oral drugs

Antiflatulants

Indications:	Relief of excess gas and bloating in the gastrointestinal tract

Simethicone (Mylicon):   Defoams gastric juice by coalescing gas bubbles

GI side effects: Effective in removal of gas, not in prevention of gas formation

Nutritional side effects: None

Interactions with other drugs: None

Antilipemics

Indications: Lower cholesterol and triglycerides in the prevention or treatment of atherosclerosis and coronary artery disease

Cholestyramine (Questran):   Increases clearance of cholesterol by binding bile acids in the gastrointestinal tract

GI side effects: Nausea, vomiting, abdominal distress, constipation and impaction, flatulence, steatorrhea

Nutritional side effects: Coordinate with restrictions in dietary intake of fat, cholesterol, and carbohydrate; increase in fiber/bulk and fluid in the diet; supplemental vitamins A, D, K, and folic acid if blood levels indicate decrease in prothrombin and folate

Interactions with other drugs: Decreases absorption of oral medications such as acetaminophen, glucocorticoids, cardiac glycosides, naproxen, ursodiol, methotrexate, phenylbutazone, propranolol, thiazide diuretics, anticoagulants, and all fat soluble vitamins (A, D, E, K); increases effect of anticoagulants

Colestipol (Colestipol):   Increases clearance of cholesterol by binding bile acids in the gastrointestinal tract

GI side effects: Same as for cholestyramine

Nutritional side effects: Same as for cholestyramine

Interactions with other drugs: Same as for cholestyramine

Clofibrate (Novofibrate):   Reduces triglycerides and very low density lipoproteins (VLDL)

GI side effects: Nausea, vomiting, abdominal distress, diarrhea, flatulence, weight gain, polyphagia, hepatitis

Interactions with other drugs: Increases effect of anticoagulants and antiprotein bound drugs such as oral hypoglycemics, furosemide

Antimicrobials

Indications: Destroy microorganisms sensitive to a specific antimicrobial in the presence of an infectious process

Penicillins-amoxicillin (Amoxil):   Bind to proteins on organism cell wall to inhibit wall synthesis

GI side effects: Nausea, vomiting, diarrhea

Nutritional side effects: None

Interactions with other drugs: Increases effect of anticoagulants; decreases effect of oral contraceptives; increases blood level if taken with probenecid

Tetracyclines-tetracycline (Achromycin):   Same as penicillins

GI side effects: Nausea, vomiting, diarrhea, esophagitis, pancreatitis

Nutritional side effects:	Decreases absorption by dietary intake of calcium, dairy foods, and iron supplements, can interfere with vitamin K synthesis
Interactions with drugs:	Increases effect of anticoagulants; decreases effect of oral contraceptives; formation of chelates with antacids, iron, calcium, and magnesium; decreases absorption with antilipemics; decreases absorption of sucralfate
Erythromycins-erythromycin (Eryc):	Same as penicillins
GI side effects:	Nausea, vomiting, abdominal discomfort, diarrhea, hepatitis
Nutritional side effects:	None
Interactions with other drugs:	Increases risk of toxicity of theophylline, cyclosporine, anticoagulants, prednisolone, alfentanil, and others
Aminoglycosides-kanamycin (Kantrex):	Same as penicillins
GI side effects:	None
Nutritional side effects:	None
Interactions with other drugs:	Decreases effect if given with penicillins; increases ototoxicity with loop diuretics; nephrotoxicity increase if given with other nephrotoxic drugs
Cephalosporins-cefaclor (Ceclor):	Same as penicillins
GI side effects:	Nausea, vomiting, abdominal cramping, diarrhea, pseudomembranous colitis

Nutritional side effects:	None
Interactions with other drugs:	Decrease in excretion by probenecid causing increase in level sulfonamides; increases effect and possible toxicity by oral hypoglycemics, anticoagulants, phenytoin methotrexate; risk of crystals in urine with methenamine and hepatitis with hepatotoxic drugs

Sulfonamides-sulfisoxazole (Gantrisin):	Interfere with folic acid synthesis needed for growth of organisms
GI side effects:	Anorexia, nausea, vomiting, hepatitis
Nutritional side effects:	Can affect folate absorption; dietary folate can be provided
Interactions with other drugs:	Decreases effectiveness of oral contraceptives, possibly estrogen; increases effectiveness of anticoagulants; increases hypoglycemia effect of sulfonylureas

Bronchodilators

Indications:	Airway bronchospasms in asthma, chronic bronchitis, chronic obstructive pulmonary disease and others to reverse obstruction
Theophylline (Theo-Dur):	Accumulates cyclic adenosine monophosphate at the beta-adrenergic (pulmonary) receptors to produce airway dilation
GI side effects:	Anorexia, nausea, vomiting, abdominal cramping

Nutritional side effects:	Increases effect by beverages containing caffeine; decreases effect by meats prepared on charcoal grill; intake of high protein and low carbohydrate diet can increase the effect and vice versa
Interactions with other drugs:	Decreases metabolism that can lead to toxicity by oral contraceptives, glucocorticoids, erythromycin, beta-adrenergic blockers, cimetidine, interferon, thiabendazole, allopurinol, and others; increases metabolism and reduces effect by phenytoin, rifampin, phenobarbital, and smoking; enhances CNS side effects of sympathomimetic agents; decreases levels by loop diuretics, isoniazid, carbamazepine
Albuterol (Ventolin):	(Same as theophylline)
Nutritional side effects:	None
Interactions with other drugs:	Decreases effect by beta-adrenergic blockers; increases side effects if taken with other adrenergics

Cardiovascular Agents

Antiarrhythmic-quinidine (Duraquin, Qinalan):	Decreases myocardial excitability and reduces conduction velocity
Indications:	Prevents atrial and ventricular arrhythmias
GI side effects:	Anorexia, bad taste in mouth, nausea, abdominal cramping, diarrhea, hepatitis
	May increase need for vitamin K
Nutritional side effects:	Limits citrus fruit juices to decrease toxicity

Interactions with other drugs:	Increases metabolism and decreases effect with phenytoin, phenobarbital, rifampin; decreases metabolism with cimetidine; increases digoxin level causing toxicity; increases action of anticoagulants and neuromuscular blocking drugs, hypotension with antihypertensives, alcohol, and nitrates; toxicity with antacids or sodium bicarbonate that cause alkaline urine, deficient vitamin K if given with anticoagulant
Inotropic-digoxin (Lanoxin):	Increases force of heart contraction and cardiac output and decreases heart rate
Indications:	Treats heart failure alone or in combination with other drugs
GI side effects:	Anorexia, nausea, vomiting, diarrhea
Nutritional side effects:	Decreases absorption by bran cereals; sodium restricted diet advised
	Potassium supplementation may be necessary
Interactions with other drugs:	Hypokalemia and risk for toxicity with thiazides and loop diuretics, glucocorticoids, amphotericin B, pipercillin; toxicity with quinidine, amiodarone, verapamil, diltiazem, cyclosporine; increases half-life if given with spironolactone; decreases absorption by antacids, antilipemics and effect of drug by thyroid drugs; cause bradycardia with beta-adrenergics and other antiarrhythmics

Anticoagulant-warfarin (Coumadin):

Prevents hepatic synthesis of vitamin K dependent clotting factors to prevent thrombosis or embolism

Indications:

Prevents or treats thrombosis, embolism, coronary occlusion

GI side effects:

Nausea, abdominal cramping

Nutritional side effects:

Effect can be antagonized by high dietary intake of foods with vitamin K content such as cabbage, broccoli, peas, liver

Interactions with other drugs:

Increases response leading to bleeding by aspirin, chloramphenicol, androgens, cefamandole, cefoperazone, cefotetan, moxalactam, urokinase, streptokinase, sulfonamides, quinidine, nonsteroid anti-inflammatory agents; decreases response by alcohol, contraceptives with estrogens, barbiturates

Cardiovascular Agents—Antihypertensives

Angiotensin converting enzyme inhibitor-captopril (Capoten):

Prevents production of angiotensin II causing stimulation of aldosterone production by blocking its conversion to an active form

Indications:

Lowers blood pressure and treats heart failure when used in combination with other drugs

GI side effects:

Anorexia, reduced taste

Nutritional side effects:

None

Interactions with other drugs:	Hypotension with antihypertensives, alcohol, phenothiazines, vasodilators; hyperkalemia with additional potassium supplements, potassium sparing diuretics; decreases effect by nonsteroid anti-inflammatory agents; decreases absorption by antacids; increased level can cause lithium or digoxin toxicity; decrease elimination and cause increased level by probenecid
Beta-adrenergic blocker-propranolol (Inderal):	Blocks stimulation of myocardial $beta_1$ and vascular $beta_2$ receptor sites
Indications:	Treats angina, hypertension given alone or with other drugs; prevents myocardial infarction
GI side effects:	Nausea, vomiting, constipation, diarrhea
Nutritional side effects:	None
Interactions with other drugs:	Bradycardia if given with cardiac glycosides; hypotension with antihypertensives, alcohol, nitrates; hypertension and bradycardia if given with cocaine, ephedrine, amphetamines, phenylephrine, epinephrine, norepinephrine; neutralizes the benefit of dopamine; decreases effect with thyroid drugs, nonsteroid anti-inflammatory agents; increases effect with cimetidine
Calcium channel blocker-Verapamil (Isoptin):	Prevents calcium transport into cardiac and vascular smooth muscle, promotes coronary vasodilation
Indications:	Treats hypertension, angina

GI side effects:	Nausea, abdominal discomfort, constipation
Nutritional side effects:	Grapefruit products consumed within 2 hours may result in hypertension
Interactions with other drugs:	Severe hypertension with fentanyl and risk for toxicity from theophylline and increase in digoxin level; risk for bradycardia, heart failure, arrhythmia with disopyramide and beta-adrenergic blocker; hypotension with additional antihypertensives, alcohol, nitrates, quinidine; decrease in effect by calcium and vitamin D given at the same time; decreases metabolism and risk for toxicity of cyclosporine, prazosin, quinidine; can affect lithium levels
Central acting adrenergic-methyldopa (Aldomet):	Stimulates central alpha adrenergic receptors that inhibit vasoconstriction resulting in decrease in peripheral resistance
Indications:	Treats moderate to severe hypertension when used alone or with other drugs
GI side effects:	Dry mouth, diarrhea
Nutritional side effects:	None
Interactions with other drugs:	Hypotension with antihypertensives, alcohol, or nitrates; decreases effect by tricyclic antidepressants, nonsteroid anti-inflammatory agents, amphetamines, phenothiazines; increases lithium toxicity

Digestants

Indications:	Treat pancreatic insufficiency by lipolytic, proteolytic, and amylolytic action
Pancrelipase (Pancrease):	Increases digestion of proteins, carbohydrates, and fats in the gastrointestinal tract
GI side effects:	Anorexia, nausea, abdominal cramping or pain, diarrhea, irritation of oral mucosa
Nutritional side effects:	Ingestion of alkaline foods can affect the enteric coating on tablets allowing the medication to be destroyed by acid in the stomach
Interactions with other drugs:	Decreases effect by antacids; decreases absorption of iron preparations if administered at the same time

Diuretics

Indications:	Mild to moderate hypertension administered alone or in combination with other drugs; treatment of heart failure, renal disease
Thiazide-chlorothiazide (Diuril):	Diuresis with increased excretion of sodium and water along with chloride, potassium, magnesium, and bicarbonate
GI side effects:	Anorexia, nausea, vomiting, abdominal cramping, hepatitis
Nutritional side effects:	Increases absorption with food intake, increases intake of foods high in potassium and magnesium; decreases intake of foods high in sodium

Interactions with other drugs:	Decreases excretion of lithium and decreases absorption by cholestyramine, hypokalemia with glucocorticoids, piperacillin, amphotericin B; decreases blood pressure with additional anti-hypertensives, alcohol, nitrates
Loop-furosemide (Lasix):	Diuresis with increased excretion of water, sodium chloride, calcium, and magnesium, prevents reabsorption of sodium and chloride by action at loop of Henle and distal renal tubule
GI side effects:	Nausea, vomiting, constipation, diarrhea
Nutritional side effects:	Increases intake of foods high in potassium, calcium and magnesium; decreases intake of foods high in sodium
Interactions with other drugs:	Same as for thiazide, and increases effect of anticoagulants
Potassium sparing-spironolactone (Aldactone):	Increases excretion of sodium, calcium, bicarbonate; conserves potassium and hydrogen ions by action at distal renal tubule to antagonize aldosterone effects
GI side effects:	Anorexia, nausea, vomiting, constipation, diarrhea, abdominal cramping, flatulence
Nutritional side effects:	Hyperkalemia can result with high intake of foods high in potassium content and salt substitutes

Interactions with other drugs:	Hyperkalemia with potassium supplements and angiotensin converting enzyme inhibitors; decreases excretion of lithium; decreases blood pressure with additional antihypertensives, alcohol, nitrates; causes renal reactions with a decrease in antihypertensive response caused by nonsteroidal anti-inflammatory agents
	May cause hyperglycemia in diabetics

Electrolytes

Indications:	Prevent or replace electrolytes in depletion or deficiency states
Calcium carbonate (Rolaids, Oscal):	Maintains nervous, skeletal and muscle function; prevents osteoporosis
GI side effects:	Nausea, vomiting, constipation
Nutritional side effects:	Decreases absorption with intake of spinach, cereals, or rhubarb; include vitamin D in dietary intake or oral supplement
Interactions with other drugs:	Decreases absorption of tetracycline if given at the same time; increase in calcium level can cause cardiac glycoside toxic response; milk-alkali syndrome can result if taken with antacids in presence of renal disease
Potassium chloride (K-Lor, K-Lyte):	Maintains acid-base balance, cardiac, skeletal and smooth muscle function; transmission of nerve impulses, renal and metabolic function; prevents potassium depletion when taking diuretics

GI side effects:	Nausea, vomiting, abdominal discomfort, diarrhea, gastric mucosa irritation or ulceration
Nutritional side effects:	Monitor intake of dietary potassium
Interactions with other drugs:	Hyperkalemia can result when given with potassium sparing diuretics or angiotensin converting enzyme inhibitors

Histamine H$_2$ Blockers

Indications:	Treat gastric ulcer or prevent duodenal ulcer, treat gastroesophageal reflux
Cimetidine (Tagamet):	Inhibits action of histamine at the H$_2$ receptor site in the parietal cells of the stomach causing a reduction in gastric acid secretion
GI side effects:	Nausea, constipation, diarrhea, hepatitis
Nutritional side effects:	May decrease iron absorption
	Alcohol and foods that are irritating to the gastric mucosa should be avoided
Interactions with other drugs:	Decreases oral absorption if taken with antacids; decreases absorption of tetracyclines, indomethacin and the effect of tocainide; effect on liver metabolism of drugs can lead to toxic levels of phenytoin, theophylline, anticoagulants, lidocaine, and possibly caffeine, quinidine, quinine, narcotics, procainamide, calcium channel blockers, oral hypoglycemics, metoprolol, some antidepressants, and others

Ranitidine (Zantac):	Inhibits action of histamine at the H_2 receptor site in the parietal cells of the stomach causing a reduction in gastric acid secretion
GI side effects:	Nausea, abdominal discomfort, constipation, diarrhea, hepatitis
Nutritional side effects:	Alcohol and foods that are irritating to the gastric mucosa should be avoided
Interactions with other drugs:	Decreases absorption if taken with antacids

Laxatives

Bulk forming-psyllium (Metamucil):	Combines with water to form bulk that will increase peristalsis and movement of feces through the bowel
Indications:	Treats chronic constipation especially if straining is not allowed
GI side effects:	Nausea, vomiting, abdominal cramping, obstruction
Nutritional side effects:	Anorexia can occur with feeling of abdominal fullness; increase fluid intake to prevent impaction; can contain sodium and sugar and cause electrolyte imbalance (potassium) with chronic use or overuse
Interactions with other drugs:	Decrease in absorption of salicylates, cardiac glycosides, and anticoagulants
Stool softener-Docusate calcium (Surfak), docusate sodium (Colace):	Softens feces by addition of water to the feces for easier passage of the mass
Indications:	Short-term use to prevent or treat mild constipation especially if straining is not allowed

GI side effects:	Abdominal cramping
Nutritional side effects:	Maintain fluid intake; can cause electrolyte imbalance with long-term use
Interactions with other drugs:	None

Stimulant-bisacodyl (Dulcolax):	Stimulates peristalsis to promote evacuation of the bowel
Indications:	Treats constipation caused by immobility, empty bowel prior to diagnostic procedures
GI side effects:	Nausea, abdominal cramping, diarrhea, rectal discomfort, excessive fluid losses (dehydration)
Nutritional side effects:	Increase fluid intake to prevent fluid imbalance; long-term use can cause electrolyte imbalance including decrease in potassium and calcium
Interactions with other drugs:	Decreases absorption of any other drugs as motility is increased; enteric coating can be destroyed if taken with antacids

Lubricant-mineral oil (Petrogalar):	Coats surface of feces to assist in passage through bowel
Indications: feces	Treats constipation by softening
GI side effects:	Seepage of oil from the rectum
Nutritional side effects:	Decrease in absorption of vitamins A, D, E, K (fat-soluble)
Interactions with other drugs:	Decreases absorption of vitamins A, D, E, K (fat-soluble)

Psychotherapeutic Agents

Antidepressants-
amitriptyline (Elavil),
imipramine (Tofranil):

Prevent re-uptake of dopamine, norepinephrine, and serotonin with sedation effect

Indications:

Treat depression with or without psychotherapy

GI side effects:

Anorexia, dry mouth, altered taste acuity, constipation, paralytic ileus, hepatitis

Nutritional side effects:

Fiber should be included in diet to prevent constipation; low-caloric fluids can offset dry mouth discomfort; can also stimulate appetite and cause weight gain

Interactions with other drugs:

Reduces therapeutic effect of antihypertensives and cause hypertension if given with clonidine; add to CNS depression by alcohol, antihistamines, narcotics, sedatives; increases levels leading to toxicity by cimetidine, oral contraceptives, phenothiazines; decreases effect with smoking

Antipsychotics-
chlorpromazine (Thorazine),
haloperidol (Haldol):

Effect dopamine action in CNS to reduce signs and symptoms of psychosis

Indications:

Treat psychoses and control extremes in behavior patterns

GI side effects:

Same as for antidepressants

Nutritional side effects:

None

Interactions with other drugs:	Hypotension with antihypertensives, nitrates, alcohol, and hypotension and tachycardia when taken with epinephrine; additional anticholinergic effect with antidepressants, antihistamines, quinidine, phenothiazines, atropine; CNS depression with alcohol, narcotics, antihistamines, sedatives; decreases effect of levodopa; results in confusion with methyldopa

Antianxiety/sedative-lorazepam (Ativan), diazepam (Valium):

Decreases CNS activity to relieve anxiety and/or promote sleep

Indications:	Short-term use for insomnia to provide sedation and moderate to high stress to relieve anxiety GI side effects
GI side effects:	Nausea, vomiting, constipation, diarrhea
Nutritional side effects:	Can increase appetite and cause weight gain
Interactions with other drugs:	CNS depression with alcohol, narcotics, antihistamines, antidepressants, sedatives; decreases effect of levodopa; decreases effect by smoking; decreases effect if taken with probenecid

Vitamins/Minerals

Indications:	Prevent or replace a deficiency if nutritional status warrants this

Multiple vitamins/minerals (Vicon-Forte, Theragran):	Include the fat-soluble vitamins A, D, E and water-soluble vitamins B complex, C, biotin, and folic acid plus minerals and/or trace elements to prevent or treat deficiencies/ supplement dietary intake
GI side effects:	None
Nutritional side effects:	None
Interactions with other drugs:	Large amounts of B complex can reduce effect of levodopa; decreases fat soluble vitamin absorption by mineral oil and antilipemics

Chapter X

Diagnostic Procedures and Laboratory Tests Related to the Gastrointestinal System and Nutrition/Diet Therapy

A.   Endoscopy Diagnostic Procedures
- Colonoscopy
- Esophagogastroduodenoscopy
- Proctosigmoidoscopy

B.   Imaging Diagnostic Procedures
- Computed Axial Tomography
- Magnetic Resonance Imaging
- Nuclear Imaging

C.   Radlology Diagnostic Procedures
- Abdominal Flat Plate
- Gallbladder Series
- Lower Gastrointestinal Series
- Upper Gastrointestinal Series

D.   Ultrasound Diagnostic Procedure

E.   Bilirubin Laboratory Tests
- Total Bilirubin
- Conjugated Bilirubin
- Unconjugated Bilirubin
- Urlnary Bilirubin
- Urinary Urobilinogen

F.   Carbohydrate Laboratory Tests
- Glucose, Serum
- Glucose, 2 Hour Postprandial
- Glucose Tolerance, Oral
- Glycosylated Hemoglobin
- Urinary Glucose
- Urinary Ketone Bodies

G.	Complete Blood Count
	Laboratory Tests
		Red Blood Cells
		Hemoglobin
		Hematocrit
		Red Cell Indices
		White Blood Cells
		Differential WBC
		Lymphocytes
H.	Electrolyte Laboratory Tests
		Bicarbonate
		Calcium
		Chloride
		Magnesium
		Phosphorus
		Potassium
		Sodium
		Anion Gap
I.	Enzyme Laboratory Tests
		Alanine Aminotransferase
		Alkaline Phosphatase
		Amylase
		Gamma-Glutamyl Transferase
		Lipase
J.	Feces Laboratory Tests
		Appearance
		Blood
		Mucus
		Pus
		Culture
		Microscopic
		Occult Blood
K.	Hormone Laboratory Tests
		Aldosterone
		Gastrin
		Thyroxine
		Triiodothyronine

Endoscopy Diagnostic Procedures

Colonoscopy

Colonoscopy involves the insertion of a flexible fiberoptic colonoscope with a light source into the anus and through the large intestine. It is performed to visualize and examine the mucosa of the bowel for diverticulosis, inflammatory disease, tumor, polyps, or identify a bleeding source. Polyps can also be removed and tissue biopsy specimens obtained for laboratory testing (cytology) to aid in diagnosis. In the higher risk older adult, this procedure is done periodically to screen for these disorders.

Nutritional implications include:

Resumption of usual dietary intake 2-4 hours following the procedure

Inclusion of fiber in the diet to promote elimination and prevent constipation

Esophagogastroduodenoscopy (EGD)

This procedure involves the insertion of a flexible scope with a light source into the mouth and advanced through the esophagus, stomach, and duodenum. It is performed to visualize and examine the mucosa of these organs for abnormalities such as inflammatory conditions, strictures, ulcers, tumor, and hiatal hernia. It is also done to determine the cause of dysphagia, identify the source of upper gastrointestinal bleeding, and perform tissue biopsy for laboratory testing (cytology) to aid in diagnosis. The procedure can be limited to the esophagus (esophagoscopy) or the stomach (gastroscopy).

Nutritional implications include:

Resumption of usual dietary intake after gag reflex returns and throat discomfort is relieved

Mouth care prior to eating to remove bad taste of topical anesthetic that can affect the taste of foods

Proctosigmoidoscopy

This procedure involves the insertion of a rigid or flexible proctoscope with a light source into the anus and advanced into the rectum and sigmoid colon. It is performed to visualize and examine the mucosa and structure of these areas for polyps, inflammation, abscess, fissure, fistula, internal hemorrhoids, and tumor. It is also done to determine the cause of diarrhea or identify a bleeding source. Polyps can be removed and tissue biopsy and other specimens obtained for laboratory testing (cytology and culture) to aid in diagnosis.

Nutritional implications include:

Resumption of any restricted dietary inclusions following the procedure

Imaging Diagnostic Procedures

Computed Axial Tomography (CAT, CT)

This procedure involves the scanning of body parts with a special x-ray machine that produces imaging based on body tissue or organ composition. The rays are transmitted through the tissue and a detector records the intensity from various angles. A computer then calculates and constructs slices in shades specific to tissues (black for air, white for bone, gray for organ tissue). The result is a pattern of densities that assist in the diagnosis of gastrointestinal inflammatory disease or tumor, and liver, gallbladder, or pancreatic pathology. It also assists to localize bleeding sites. An iodinated contrast medium is usually used in CT scanning of the gastrointestinal system to enhance views of organ structures.

Nutritional implications include:

Resumption of diet following the study, if side effects caused by contrast media are absent

Magnetic Resonance Imaging (MRI)

This procedure involves the scanning of body parts by a special magnetic resonance machine that provides signals based on the type and pathology of the tissue examined. The signals from the various planes are converted by a computer and portrayed on a screen for diagnostic evaluation. The procedure is noninvasive and done to diagnose and differentiate malignant from benign tumors.

Nutritional implications include:

None

Nuclear Imaging

Nuclear imaging involves the scanning of organs by equipment that detects the presence of gamma rays emitted by radionuclides specific to the system to be studied, administered prior to the procedure. The imaging reveals the size, structure, position, and function of an organ (liver, gallbladder, pancreas). It is performed to diagnose tumors and inflammatory conditions as well as other abnormalities specific to the organ to be imaged.

Nutritional implications Include:

None

Radiology Diagnostic Procedures

Abdominal Flat Plate (KUB)

This procedure involves the filming of abdominal organs to visualize size, location, and structure of the liver, gallbladder, spleen, kidneys, ureters, and bladder. It is done as a screen to detect abnormalities prior to more extensive studies to diagnose masses, obstruction, or foreign bodies of the gastrointestinal tract.

Nutritional implications include:

None

Gallbladder Series (OGB)

This procedure involves the filming of the gallbladder following the oral ingestion of iodinated contrast tablets to view organ function, inflammation, tumor, possible presence of gallstones, and cystic duct obstruction. Films are taken at intervals in varied positions to determine both filling and emptying of the gallbladder. A fat drink or diet can be given during the procedure to cause bladder contraction and subsequent filming of gallbladder function.

Nutritional implications include:

Resumption of food and fluids following completion of the study

Lower Gastrointestinal Series (LGI)

This procedure involves the filming and fluoroscopic viewing of the large intestine in various positions following the administration of a barium contrast medium enema. It is performed to determine the position and shape of the colon, and to assist in the diagnosis of diverticulosis, tumor, inflammatory disorders, polyps, and obstruction.

Nutritional implications include:

Resumption of dietary and fluid intake following the study

Laxatives for 1-2 days following the study to clear the colon of barium

Upper Gastrointestinal Series (UGI)

This procedure involves the filming and fluoroscopic viewing of the esophagus, stomach, and small bowel following the administration of a barium contrast medium swallow. It is performed to determine the size, shape, position, and movement of the barium through these organs and the diagnosis of hiatal hernia, peptic ulcer, diverticula of the stomach or duodenum tumor, inflammatory conditions, esophageal varices or strictures.

Nutritional implications include:

Resumption of dietary and fluid intake following the study

Laxatives if needed to clear the barium from the gastrointestinal tract

Ultrasound Diagnostic Procedure

Ultrasonography (Echography, Sonography)

This procedure involves the soft tissue visualization of organs (gallbladder, biliary system, liver, pancreas) with the use of high frequency sound waves that pass through the body and are recorded on a screen (oscilloscope) as they are echoed or bounced back. It can be performed to detect peristaltic movement and differences in tissue densities from normal tissue to reveal masses, liver cirrhosis, gallstones and biliary obstruction, and pancreatic tumor. Abnormalities are usually confirmed by nuclear imaging or computerized tomography.

Nutritional implications include:

Resumption of dietary and fluid intake, if restricted, following the study

Bilirubin Laboratory Tests	Chemistry
Total Bilirubin	0.1-1.0 mg/dL
Conjugated Bilirubin (Direct)	0-0.3 mg/dL
Unconjugated Bilirubin (Indirect)	0.1-0.8 mg/dL
Urinary Bilirubin	Negative
Urinary Urobilinogen	0.1-1.0 Ehrlich unit/dL (Random)
	Adult female: 0.1-1.1 Ehrlich units (2 Hr)
	Adult male: 0.3-2.1 Ehrlich units (2 Hr)

Bilirubin is a product of the destruction of RBCs produced in the liver. Total bilirubin consists of conjugated, or direct, that is excreted via the intestine; and unconjugated, or indirect, that is found in the blood circulation to the liver and excreted in the bile. Jaundice results when bilirubin reaches levels that cause it to move into tissues and leave a yellowish color. Total bilirubin level will increase with any jaundice but conjugated and unconjugated bilirubin increases are related to specific diseases. In the older adult, total bilirubin can be included in routine blood testing and total and conjugated tests are the types more commonly done. Increased total levels can indicate alcoholic, infectious, or obstructive hepatitis. An increase in total bilirubin can lead to examination for conjugated and unconjugated levels for a more specific diagnosis. Conjugated increases can indicate cirrhosis, hepatitis, biliary obstruction, or head of the pancreas tumor; unconjugated increases can indicate pernicious anemia or any type of hepatitis.

Urine can also be tested to screen for conjugated bilirubin and urobilinogen. Bilirubin can be present in hepatic or obstructive jaundice which results in bilirubin being present in the blood stream for excretion by the renal system, instead of the gastrointestinal tract for excretion in the bowel. The part of urobilinogen not excreted in the feces is reabsorbed into the blood stream, circulated to the liver and excreted in the bile or carried to the kidneys and excreted in the urine. Increased levels are found in hepatic or biliary disorders that cause decreases of urobilinogen in the bile and increases in the urine. These tests can be performed by laboratory analysis or dipstick methods.

Carbohydrate Laboratory Tests	Normal Values
Glucose, serum (FBG)	Adult: 70-110 mg/dL
Glucose, 2 Hour Postprandial	Adult: < 140 mg/dL
Glucose Tolerance, oral (GTT)	30 minutes: 150-160 mg/dL
	1 hour: 160-170 mg/dL
	1 1/2 hours: 145-155 mg/dL
	2 hours: < 140 mg/dL

Carbohydrate Laboratory Tests	Chemistry (Nationwide Standards Per Day)
Glycosylated Hemoglobin (GHB) (HbA_{1C})	Nondiabetic: 3.0%-6.0% Hb
	Diabetic: 7.0%-11.0% Hb
Urinary Glucose	Negative (Random)
Urinary Ketone Bodies (Acetone)	Negative (Random)

Carbohydrate tests are primarily done to diagnose diabetes mellitus or to determine the status of the disease. Glucose is the main source of energy in the body, and serum glucose is done to detect abnormalities in carbohydrate metabolism. This is most commonly caused by a decrease or absence of insulin production by the pancreas. The more specific tests for diabetes mellitus are the glucose tolerance test that is performed following fasting glucose levels of 126 mg/dL. The disease is confirmed by this test if glucose levels are higher than normal 1-2 hours after ingestion of glucose and are slower to return to expected normal levels. The 2 hour postprandial glucose is done to confirm a diagnosis of diabetes if normal levels are not attained 2 hours following a test meal or to evaluate the more immediate control status of diabetes. Glycosylated hemoglobin evaluates the long-term (4 month) control status of the disease. Glucose is bound to hemoglobin and the amount of glycosylated hemoglobin in the RBC depends on the available glucose for the life of the RBC, usually 4 months. Increased percentage levels of Hb indicate a hyperglycemic state during the period prior to the test.

Urinary glucose and ketone bodies testing on random specimens are done to determine the presence of these substances in evaluating diabetes. Routine urinary glucose testing is performed by dipstick (enzyme test) or Clinitest (reduction test) to monitor for glucosuria in the treatment and control of the disease. Routine testing for ketone bodies is performed by dipstick to determine the accumulation of these substances. This occurs when stored carbohydrates are absent and stored triglycerides are broken down. Both tests can also be performed by laboratory analysis.

Complete Blood Count (CBC) Laboratory Tests	**Hematology**
Red Blood Cells (RBC)	Adult female: 4.0-5.3 million/mm^3
	Adult male: 4.4-6.0 million/mm^3
	Older adult: 3-5 million/mm^3
Hemoglobin (Hb)	Adult female: 12-16 g/dL
	Adult male: 13-18 g/dL
	Older adult: 10-17 g/dL
Hematocrit (Hct)	Adult female: 37-48% or 37-48 g/dL
	Adult male: 45-52% or 45-52 g/dL
Red Cell Indices:	
Mean Corpuscular Volume (MCV)	Adult female: 81-99 μm^3
	Adult male: 80-94 μm^3
Mean Corpuscular Hemoglobin (MCH)	Adult female: 27-31 pg
Mean Corpuscular Hemoglobin Concentration (MCHC)	Adult female: 32-36%
White Blood Cells (WBC):	5,000-10,000/mm^3
Differential WBC:	
Basophils	0-1% or 25-100/mm^3
Eosinophils	1-4% or 50-400/mm^3
Neutrophils	54-75% or 3,000-7,500/mm^3
Lymphocytes:	25-40% or 1,500-4,500/mm^3
T-cells	60-80% of Lymphocytes
B-cells	10-20% of Lymphocytes
Platelets	150,000-450,000/mm^3

In general, there is a decline in RBCs for both sexes in the older adult. The RBC transports oxygen from the lungs to all organs and tissues and removes carbon dioxide from the tissues to the organs for excretion. This is achieved via its Hb component, the main intracellular protein of the RBC. The RBC, Hb, and Hct determinations are important in the diagnosis of anemia, blood loss, and in diseases affecting erythropoiesis, if levels are decreased; increased levels are found in dehydration, the polycythemias, and in some chronic diseases. Hct normally parallels the RBC and is usually three times the Hb level. Red cell indices reflect the size, weight, and content of the RBCs and their determinations are useful in diagnosing the different types of anemias.

WBC count provides information about a general body response to pathology. The differential count provides a more definitive diagnosis of infectious or inflammatory disease and immune or auto-immune disorders.

A platelet count provides information about numbers necessary for hemostasis, and platelet function is determined by other tests such as bleeding time, platelet aggregation, and platelet survival time. Both are important to protect the body against blood loss.

Although the CBC is usually performed routinely as a panel of blood cell tests, each test can be performed individually when information is desired about one specific test.

Electrolyte Laboratory Tests   Chemistry

Bicarbonate (HCO_3)	22-26 mEq/L
Calcium (Ca)	4.5-5.5 mEq/L (Total)
	2.2-2.5 mEq/L (Ionized)
Chloride (Cl)	95-105 mEq/L
Magnesium (Mg)	1.5-2.5 mEq/L
Phosphorus (PO_4)	2.4-4.5 mg/dL
Potassium (K)	3.5-5.0 mEq/L
Sodium (Na)	135-145 mEq/L
Anion Gap	7-17 mEq/L

Electrolyte testing can be performed as a panel to screen for alteration in fluid and electrolyte balance, and acid-base balance. They are substances that become ions when dissolved in body fluid. The most important ones are Na+, K+, Cl-, and HCO_3- -. Electrolyte balance and amounts are controlled by the exchange of oxygen and carbon dioxide in the lungs, kidney function in the absorption, secretion, and excretion of substances, and the endocrine gland secretion of hormones that regulate the body functions.

Testing of individual electrolytes can also be performed and increases or decreases are associated with many possible disorders and drug regimens.

Enzyme Laboratory Tests	Chemistry
Alanine Aminotransferase (ALT, SGPT)	Adult female: 4-35 U/L Adult male: 7-45 U/L
Alkaline Phosphatase (ALP)	Adult: 20-90 U/L
Amylase	Adult: 80-180 Somogyi U/dL
Gamma Glutamyl Transferase (GGT)	Adult female: 6-37 U/L Adult male: 6-37 U/L
Lipase	Adult: 14-280 U/L

Enzymes are catalysts in the body that are available for all reactions; they also maintain normal function of the organs. Those listed are related to organs and tissues such as the liver, pancreas, gallbladder, parotid glands, and duodenum. Alterations in specific organ tissues that allow enzymes to escape into the circulating blood reveal increases indicating abnormal function associated with a disease process. Tests for specific enzymes are performed when disorders of the liver, pancreas, gallbladder, biliary tract, or the digestive process are suspected. These can include injury, tumor, inflammation or obstruction involving these body organs and functions.

Feces Laboratory Tests	Feces/Microbiology
Appearance (Random)	Amount: About 100-200 g/24 hours
	Color: Brown
	Odor: Varies with pH (slightly alkaline)
	Consistency: Soft to bulky to dry and formed
Blood	Negative
Mucus	Negative
Pus	Negative
Culture	Normal flora
Microscopic:	
Fat	Fatty Acids: 5-15%
	Triglycerides: 1-5%
WBC	Negative
Epithelial Cells	Few
Parasites	Negative
Occult Blood	Negative or 5-7% of dietary intake

Routine feces analysis is a common screening test done to detect the appearance and constituents associated with gastrointestinal disorders. This test is done on a random specimen and includes amount, color, odor, consistency, and gross blood, mucus or pus. It also includes microscopic examination for fat, abnormal cells and parasites. The test for occult blood can be done by laboratory analysis or guaiac testing to determine gastrointestinal bleeding. Feces culture is a microbiological examination done on a random specimen to determine a possible enteric bacterial cause of severe diarrhea.

Hormone Laboratory Tests	Chemistry
Aldosterone	Adult female: 5-30 ng/dL
	Adult male: 6-22 ng/dL
Gastrin	Adult: 50-150 pg/ml (increases >60 yrs)
Thyroxine (T$_4$)	Adult female >60: 5.5-10.5 µgdL
	Adult male >60: 5.0-10.0 µgdL
Triiodothyronine (T$_3$)	Adult: 80-200 ng/dL

These substances control activities of related tissues and their effects are exerted at the release sites or distant sites. They act by changing the synthesis and secretion of other hormones and enzymes including the rate of enzyme activity. Their secretion is controlled by the body's need to accomplish a specific hormonal function. Following a reduction in the activity of a hormone, a negative feedback is decreased and the rate of hormone secretion is increased. Aldosterone is released to increase fluid volume and prevent fluid deficit in response to decreased sodium levels. Gastrin is associated with abnormal gastric conditions related to gastric acid production. Thyroid hormones increase the metabolic activities of tissues that result in increased oxygen use and utilization of carbo-hydrates, proteins, fats, and vitamins. These specific tests are performed when fluid or metabolic disorders that affect nutritional status are suspected.

Lipid Laboratory Tests	Chemistry
Cholesterol	Adult >50: 170-265 mg/dL
Lipoproteins:	
High Density Lipoprotein (HDL)	Adult >50: 34-75 mg/dL
Low Density Lipoprotein (LDL)	Adult >50: 105-200 mg/dL
Triglycerides	Adult female: 10-180 mg/dL
	Adult male: 10-190 mg/dL

These substances are compounds that are sources of energy needed for metabolic activities. They are derived from dietary intake and body processes. Fats in the diet (animal and plant sources) are triglycerides composed of fatty acids and glycerol with small amounts of cholesterol (animal sources) and other lipids. The body is also able to produce fats. Glucose and amino acids can be converted to fatty acids in the liver, and phospholipids and cholesterol can be produced in the liver or intestine. Lipoproteins are formed in the liver, exist in the blood, and are classified by their density. The lowest density indicates the highest triglyceride level and vice versa. These tests are done to assist in the diagnosis of abnormal liver function, atherosclerosis, and coronary artery disease.

Mineral/Vitamin Laboratory Tests	Chemistry
Vitamins:	
Vitamin A	65-275 IU/dL
Vitamin C	0.2-2.0 mg/dL
Vitamin D	0.7-3.3 IU/mL
Vitamin E	0.8-1.8 mg/dL
Trace Minerals:	
Copper (Cu)	130-230 mg/dL
Iodine (I)	4-8 mg/dL
Zinc (Zn)	50-150 mg/dL
Iron Tests:	
Ferritin	Adult female: 12-150 µg/L
	Adult male: 15-300 µg/L
Iron (Fe)	Adult female: 40-150 µg/dL
	Adult male: 50-160 µg/dL
Transferrin	200-400 mg/dL
Total Iron-Binding Capacity (TIBC)	250-400 µg/dL

Vitamins are substances involved in metabolic functions. They are supplied by dietary intake, since they cannot be synthesized by the body. They are measured to assist in the diagnosis of vitamin deficiencies. Trace minerals are also essential to normal body function. Copper promotes absorption of iron from the intestine and is essential in hemoglobin formation and other functions. Iodine is essential for thyroid hormone synthesis. Zinc, as a component of specific enzymes, assists with protein and carbohydrate metabolism. Iron is a component of hemoglobin, and iron and related tests are done to diagnose iron deficiency anemia. Other trace minerals in minute amounts are cobalt, manganese, chromium and molybdenum.

Protein Laboratory Tests	Chemistry
Proteins:	
Albumin	3.3-4.5 g/dL
Globulin	2.0-4.2 g/dL
Albumin/Globulin Ratio (A/G)	1.5:1.0-2.5:1.0
Total Proteins	6.6-7.9 g/dL
Protein Metabolites:	
Ammonia	15-45 µg/dL
Blood Urea Nitrogen (BUN)	6-20 mg/dL

Proteins consist of amino acids linked together by peptide chains. Amino acids are provided from dietary intake, and are distributed to cells and incorporated into proteins. Plasma proteins include albumin, globulins, and fibrinogen. These proteins in the blood transport amino acids for synthesis and metabolic processes. These tests provide a screening of protein homeostasis and can be included in multi-testing chemistry panels. Amino acid profiles reflect a deficiency in any single essential amino acid. Changes in protein levels can result from dehydration, nutritional deficiencies, malabsorption problems, diarrhea or vomiting, as well as more acute conditions involving the liver, renal or other system dysfunctions. Protein metabolites are end-products of protein metabolism and reflects protein metabolism and balance. Abnormal levels of these substances indicate liver (ammonia) or renal (BUN) impairment.

Schilling Laboratory Tests	Nuclear
24 Hour Urine Analysis	>10% of dose excreted
Pernicious anemia	<2% of dose excreted

This test is performed on a 24 hour urine specimen following an oral dose of a vitamin B_{12} tagged with a radionuclide and intramuscular injection of vitamin B_{12}. The injection is administered to saturate all the binding sites and enhance excretion of the radionuclide. It is done to diagnose pernicious anemia. The absence of intrinsic factor of the stomach in this disease prevents absorption of the oral vitamin, resulting in an absence of or limited amounts of urinary excretion. The urine is examined for the percentage of radioactive B_{12} dosage excreted to determine the presence of this deficiency.

Urine Laboratory Tests	Urine/Microbiology
Appearance (Random)	Color: Yellow to amber depending on sp. gr.
	Turbidity: Clear to slightly cloudy
	Odor: Faint aroma
Blood (Hematuria)	Negative
Culture (Mid-stream specimen)	Negative for pathogens
Microscopic:	
RBC	0-3 per high power field
WBC	0-4 per high power field
Epithelial Cells	Few
Casts	Occasional
Crystals	Occasional

Urine Laboratory Tests	*Urine Microbiology*
Nitrite	Negative
Osmolality	500-850 mOsm/kg H_2O
pH	4.5-8.0
Specific Gravity (sp. gr.)	1.001-1.035
Glucose, Protein, Ketones, Bilirubin, and Urobilinogen	Included in related test groups

Routine urinalysis is a common screening test done to detect abnormal constituents and appearance associated with disorders of the renal system, and possible fluid imbalance. This test is performed on a random specimen and includes color, clarity, pH, sp. gr., nitrite for bacteria, glucose, ketones, protein, bilirubin, urobilinogen, and blood determinations. It also includes microscopic examination of sediment for abnormal cells, casts, and crystals. The test for osmolality reveals a more accurate determination of urine concentration and sp. gr. Urine culture is a microbiological test done on a clean mid-stream specimen to determine the presence of a urinary tract infection with a count of > 100,000 bacteria /mL.

APPENDIX

ABBREVIATIONS

BP	Blood Pressure	NANDA	North American Nursing Diagnosis Association
C	Centigrade/Celsius	N/G	Nasogastric
CDC	Center for Disease Control	NPO	Nothing by mouth
CNS	Central Nervous System	P	Pulse
cu	Cubic	PO	Orally
cm	Centimeter	R	Respiration
F	Farenheit	RDA	Recommended Daily Allowance
g	Gram	sec	Second
GI	Gastrointestinal	T	Temperature
h	Hour	TPN	Total Parenteral Nutrition
HCl	Hydrochloric Acid	VS	Vital Signs
Ht	Height	wk	Week
IM	Intramuscular	μg	Microgram
I&O	Intake and Output	Wt	Weight
IV	Intravenous	<	Less than
kg	Kilogram	>	More than
lb	Pound		
Liter	Liter		
mEq	Milliequivalent/Per		
mg	Milligram		
mL	Milliliter		
min	Minute		
mm	Millimeter		

GLOSSARY

Absorption:
>The process associated with the passage of nutrients through the intestinal mucosa

Acid:
>A substance that releases hydrogen ions (H+) and with a pH

Acidosis:
>An increase of acid with a decrease in alkali in the blood

Alkalosis:
>A deficit of acid or an accumulation of alkali in the blood

Amino Acids:
>The units that make up proteins

Anabolism:
>The process that metabolizes nutrients into complex substances for cell building and maintenance

Anion:
>An electrolyte with a negative charge

Anorexia:
>Lack of appetite

Base:
>A substance that accepts the hydrogen ion

Bolus:
>A food mass produced in the mouth and passed through the esophagus

Cachexia:
>An emaciated state of nutritional deficit associated with chronic illness

Calorie:
>The amount of heat or energy that raises the temperature of a gram of water 1 degree C

Carbohydrate:
> A substance composed of hydrogen, carbon and oxygen called a starch

Caries:
> The process of tooth decay

Catabolism:
> The process that metabolizes nutrients into smaller substances that is destructive to cell structure

Cation:
> An electrolyte with a positive charge

Cellulose:
> A part of plants that is not digestible by humans

Chyme:
> The food that is liquified during the process of digestion

Complex Protein:
> A protein that contains all of the essential proteins necessary for growth and maintenance of cells

Dehydration:
> An excess of fluid loss

Digestion:
> The process of the breakdown of foods to a form that can be absorbed by the gastrointestinal tract

Disaccharides:
> The linkage of two monosaccharides

Dysphagia:
> Difficult swallowing

Electrolyte:
> A substance that dissociates into ions when dissolved in water

Emesis:
> Vomiting

Enteral Feeding:
>Introducing nutrients into the gastrointestinal tract via a tube

Enzyme:
>A substance that acts as a catalyst for chemical reactions in the body

Essential Amino Acids:
>An amino acid that is not synthesized by the body and must be secured through dietary intake

Essential Fatty Acids:
>The polyunsaturated fats that are not synthesized by the body and must be secured through dietary intake

Excretion:
>The process of waste elimination from the body

Fat:
>A substance composed of carbon, oxygen, and hydrogen in water

Fatty Acids:
>The components of fats classified according to number of carbons and bonds between them

Fiber:
>The carbohydrate portion in plants and meats that cannot be digested by humans, also called bulk in the diet

Geriatric:
>The specialty in medicine concerned with diseases in the aged population

Gerontology:
>The study of aging

Globulin:
>A protein found in the blood plasma important in fighting infection

Glucose:
>A monosaccharide found in the blood available for immediate use and energy, also called dextrose

Glyceride:
>   The simplest form of lipid consisting of glycerol and one or more fatty acids

Hormone:
>   A substance produced by an endocrine gland that regulates body functions

Hypertonic:
>   A fluid with higher osmolarity than body fluid

Hypotonic:
>   A fluid with lower osmolarity than body fluid

Hypogeusia:
>   Loss of taste sensation

Hyposmia:
>   Loss of smell sensation

Ingestion:
>   The process of eating or drinking

Ion:
>   An atom with a positive or negative charge

Isotonic:
>   A fluid with the same osmolarity as body fluid

Lipids:
>   Fat and fat related substances

Malnutrition:
>   An over or under nutritional state

Mastication:
>   Chewing or grinding food

Metabolism:
>   The total of all chemical processes in the body, anabolism and catabolism

Milk-Alkali Syndrome:
>   Excessive intake of milk and an alkali resulting in alkalosis and renal dysfunction

Milliequivalent:
>A unit of measurement derived from the atomic weight of a substance divided by the valence of a substance

Minerals:
>Part of the body composition and the inorganic parts of food that are necessary for body function

Monosaccharides:
>A simple sugar that cannot be broken down by hydrolysis

Nitrogen Balance:
>Equality of nitrogen intake and excretion

Nonessential Amino Acids:
>An amino acid that can be synthesized by the body

Nutrient:
>A substance in food that can be ingested, digested, absorbed, and utilized by the body

Osmosis:
>Movement of a solvent through a membrane from a less concentrated to a more concentrated solution

Peristalsis:
>The contraction and relaxation of the muscles of the gastrointestinal tract that moves a food bolus

Polysaccharide:
>A combination of monosaccharide units (10 or more)

Proteins:
>A nitrogen containing organic compound composed of amino acids

Regurgitation:
>Reflux of swallowed food into the mouth

Senescence:
>The process of aging or being elderly

Synthesis:
>The combination of substances to build or form a new substance

Triglyceride:
> A combination of three fatty acids and glycerol, also called a fat

Vitamins:
> Substances found in foods that are necessary to perform specific functions in metabolism

NUTRITION AND HEALTH RESOURCES

American Association of Retired Persons
601 East Street, NW
Washington, DC 20049
(202) 434-3680

American Geriatrics Society
Suite 300
770 Lexington Avenue
New York, NY 10021
(212) 308-1414

American Dietetic Association
Suite 800
216 West Jackson Boulevard
Chicago, IL 60606
(312) 899-0040

Administration on Aging
330 Independence Avenue, SW
Washington, DC 20201
(202) 619-0724

Center for Nutrition Policy and Promotion
1120 20th Street, NW
Suite 200, North Lobby
Washington, DC 20036
(202) 418-2312

National Institute on Aging
Public Information Office
Federal Building, Room 6C12
9000 Rockville Pike
Bethesda, MD 20892
(301) 496-1752

Office of Disease Prevention and Health Promotion
National Health Information Center
PO Box 1133
Washington, DC 20013-1133
1 (800) 336-4797

USDA Food and Nutrition Service
Office of Government Affairs/Public Information
3101 Park Center Dr., Room 805
Alexandria, VA 22302-1594
(703) 305-2031

REFERENCES

American Diabetes Association. *Exchange Lists for Meal Planning.* Diabetes Information Service Center. Alexandria, VA, 1995.

American Diabetes Association. *Month of Meals Menu Planner,* vol 1–5. Diabetes Information Service Center. Alexandria, VA, 1989-94.

American Dietetic Association. *Nutrition Interventions Manual for Professionals Caring for Older Americans.* Chicago, 1991.

Black, JM and Matassarin-Tacobs, E. *Luckmann and Sorensen's Medical-Surgical Nursing: A Psychophysiologic Approach* (4th ed.). Philadephia: WB Saunders, 1993.

Chernecky, CC, et al. *Laboratory Tests and Diagnostic Procedures* (2nd ed.). Philadephia: WB Saunders, 1997.

Davis, J and Sherer, K. *Applied Nutrition and Diet Therapy for Nurses* (2nd ed.). Philadelphia: WB Saunders, 1994.

Deglin, TH and Vallerand, AH. *Davis's Drug Guide for Nurses* (5th ed.). Philadelphia: FA Davis, 1997.

Doenges, ME and Moorhouse, MF. *Nurse's Pocket Guide: Nursing Diagnoses with Interventions* (6th ed.). Philadelphia: FA Davis, 1997.

Feldman, EB. *Essentials of Clinical Nutrition.* Philadelphia: FA Davis, 1988.

Kim, MJ, et al. *Pocket Guide to Nursing Diagnoses* (7th ed.). St. Louis: Mosby-Year Book, 1997.

LaQuatra, IM and Gerlach, MJ. *Nutrition in Clinical Nursing.* Albany: Delmar Publishers, 1990.

Mahan, LK and Arlin, M. *Krause's Food, Nutrition and Diet Therapy* (9th ed.). Philadelphia: WB Saunders, 1996.

Moore, MC. *Pocket Guide to Nutrition and Diet Therapy.* St. Louis: Mosby-Year Book, 1992.

North American Nursing Diagnosis Association. *Taxonomy I - Revised with Official Nursing Diagnoses.* St. Louis: Tenth National Conference, 1992.

Rhodes, SS. *Effective Menu Planning for the Elderly Nutrition Program.* Chicago: The American Dietetic Association, 1991.

Schlenker, ED. *Nutrition in Aging* (3rd ed.). St. Louis: Mosby-Year Book, 1997.

U.S. Department of Health & Human Services. National Institutes of Health, No 94-3680, 1993.

Williams, SR. *Essentials of Nutrition and Diet Therapy* (6th ed.). St. Louis: Mosby-Year Book, 1994.

Williams, SR, et al. *Nutrition Throughout the Life Cycle* (2nd ed.). St. Louis: Mosby-Year Book, 1992.

Skidmore-Roth Publishing, Inc. Order Form

Qty	Title	Price	Total
	Geriatric Nursing Care Plans (2nd ed.), Jaffe 1996	$38.95	
	Geriatric Survival Handbook (3rd ed.), Acello 1997	$26.95	
	Geriatric Long-Term Procedures and Treatments (2nd ed.), Jaffe 1994	$34.95	
	Geriatric Outline, Morice 1995	$23.95	
	Body in Brief (3rd ed.), Rayman 1997	$35.95	
	Diagnostic and Lab Cards (3rd ed.), Skidmore-Roth 1998	$28.95	
	Drug Comparison Handbook (2nd ed.), Reilly 1995	$35.95	
	Nurse's Trivia Calendar, Rayman	$12.95	

Prices subject to change without notice. Shipping and handling will be added. CO residents add sales tax.	Subtotal	
	CO Sales Tax	
	S & H	
	Total	

Name

Company

Address   City

State   Zip   Phone

____ Check enclosed   ____ Visa   ____ Mastercard

Credit Card Number

Card Holder Name

Signature   Exp Date

For fastest service call 1-800-825-3150. Orders are accepted by mail with payment.

Skidmore-Roth Publishing, Inc.
400 Inverness Drive South
Suite 260
Englewood, Colorado 80112
1-800-825-3150

Visit our website at: http://www.skidmore-roth.com